Ten Teachers'
Self-assessment in
Gynaecology and
Obstetrics

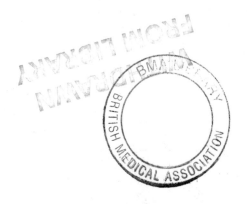

BRITISH MEDICAL ASSOCIATION

1004708

TEN TEACHERS' SELF-ASSESSMENT IN GYNAECOLOGY AND OBSTETRICS

MULTIPLE-CHOICE AND SHORT-ANSWER QUESTIONS

FOURTH EDITION

Marcus E. Setchell MA, FRCS, FRCOG

Consultant Obstetrician and Gynaecologist,
Whittington Hospital, London; Honorary Senior Lecturer,
University College of London; Honorary Consultant,
St Bartholomew's and Homerton Hospitals, London

AND

Basky Thilaganathan MD, MRCOG

Senior Lecturer and Director, Fetal Medicine Unit,
St George's Hospital Medical School, London

A member of the Hodder Headline Group
LONDON • NEW YORK • NEW DELHI

BMA LIBRARY
WITHDRAWN FROM
BRITISH MEDICAL ASSOCIATION

First published in Great Britain in 2001 by
Arnold, a member of the Hodder Headline Group,
338 Euston Road, London NW1 3BH

http://www.arnoldpublishers.com

Distributed in the USA by
Oxford University Press Inc.,
198 Madison Avenue, New York, NY10016
Oxford is a registered trademark of Oxford University Press

© 2001 Marcus Setchell and Basky Thilaganathan

All rights reserved. No part of this publication may be reproduced or
transmitted in any form or by any means, electronically or mechanically,
including photocopying, recording or any information storage or retrieval
system, without either prior permission in writing from the publisher or a
licence permitting restricted copying. In the United Kingdom such licences
are issued by the Copyright Licensing Agency: 90 Tottenham Court Road,
London W1T 4LP.

Whilst the advice and information in this book are believed to be true and
accurate at the date of going to press, neither the author[s] nor the publisher
can accept any legal responsibility or liability for any errors or omissions
that may be made. In particular (but without limiting the generality of the
preceding disclaimer) every effort has been made to check drug dosages;
however, it is still possible that errors have been missed. Furthermore,
dosage schedules are constantly being revised and new side-effects
recognized. For these reasons the reader is strongly urged to consult the
drug companies' printed instructions before administering any of the drugs
recommended in this book.

British Library Cataloguing in Publication Data
A catalogue record for this book is available from the British Library

Library of Congress Cataloging-in-Publication Data
A catalog record for this book is available from the Library of Congress

ISBN 0 340 76068 0

1 2 3 4 5 6 7 8 9 10

Commissioning Editor: Georgina Bentliff
Editorial Assistant: Zoë Elliott
Production Editor: Wendy Rooke
Production Controller: Bryan Eccleshall
Design and Typesetting by J&L Composition Ltd, Filey, North Yorkshire
Printed and bound in India by Replika Press PVT Ltd

What do you think about this book? Or any other Arnold title?
Please send your comments to feedback.arnold@hodder.co.uk

Contents

TEN TEACHERS' SELF-ASSESSMENT

TEN TEACHERS' SELF-ASSESSMENT

Preface

When this volume was first published in 1985, multiple-choice questions had only recently become an established part of undergraduate clinical examinations. Time has moved on, and in addition to MCQs, many universities now include structured short answers in their examinations.

The aim of the original book was to allow students to test their own knowledge against their reading, as well as to provide practice for their examination in Obstetrics and Gynaecology.

Ten Teachers in Obstetrics and Gynaecology were the textbooks on which all of the questions were based. With the acquisition of a completely new set of authors, as well as editors, these long-established student textbooks have recently had their most radical revision ever. It is therefore fitting that *Ten Teachers' Self-Assessment in Gynaecology and Obstetrics* should have a new author to bring about a comparable radical revision. We have updated and expanded the number of multiple-choice questions, and we have regrouped them in line with the chapters in the new *Ten Teachers*, and introduced 30 short-answer questions.

We are sad to say farewell to Professor Richard Lilford, who was one of the authors for the first three editions of this book. He has now moved away from clinical practice and education to Research and Development Management. This has made way for Mr Basky Thilaganathan, Senior Lecturer at St George's Hospital, who has provided a very welcome new perspective and fresh ideas.

We are, as ever, grateful to the authors of *Ten Teachers*, whose writing has stimulated the questions, to colleagues who have made helpful comments on the questions, and to the publishers for their forbearance.

Marcus E. Setchell
Basky Thilaganathan

CHAPTER ONE

Gynaecology MCQs

EMBRYOLOGY, ANATOMY AND PHYSIOLOGY

1 During development of the genital organs:

   (a) The genital organs develop from the ectoderm
   (b) The paramesonephric duct develops to form the Müllerian system
   (c) The Müllerian duct divides to form the Fallopian tubes and ovaries
   (d) The genital tubercle forms the clitoris and labia majora
   (e) The number of oocytes starts to decline from before birth

2 The nerve supply to the vulva is derived from:

   (a) The pudendal nerve
   (b) The ilio-inguinal nerve
   (c) The genitofemoral nerve
   (d) The posterior cutaneous nerve of the thigh
   (e) The inferior haemorrhoidal nerve

3 The support of the uterus is provided by:

   (a) The cardinal ligaments
   (b) The round ligaments
   (c) The utero-sacral ligaments
   (d) The integrity of the perineal body
   (e) The broad ligament

4 The internal reproductive organs:

   (a) The vagina is lined with skin (stratified squamous epithelium)
   (b) Vaginal Döderlein's bacilli convert glycogen to keep the pH above 7.5
   (c) The epithelium of the cervix is partly squamous and partly ciliated
   (d) The isthmus of the Fallopian tube is the most medial portion
   (e) The ovary is covered by a thin layer of peritoneum

5 Age changes in the genital tract:

   (a) There is increased atrophy and fat deposition in the vulva after the
        menopause
   (b) The vagina is devoid of glycogen before puberty and after the
        menopause
   (c) The ratio of cervical to uterine length decreases after the menopause
   (d) Remnants of the hymen after childbirth are known as carunculae
        myrtiformes
   (e) At birth, the neonatal vagina is well developed and has a low pH (< 5)

1 (a) **False** They develop from the mesoderm.
   (b) **True** The mesonephric duct develops into the Wolffian (male) system.
   (c) **False** The Müllerian ducts fuse to form a single uterus.
   (d) **False** The labia majora form from the genital folds.
   (e) **True** At birth, there are 2 million germ cells, half of which are atretic.

2 (a) **True** The pudendal nerve (S2,3,4) gives off the inferior rectal branch before dividing into the perineal and dorsal nerves of the clitoris.
   (b) **True** The ilio-inguinal and genitofemoral nerves supply sensory fibres.
   (c) **True** To the mons and labia.
   (d) **True** It carries some sensory fibres to the perineum.
   (e) **False** This branch of the pudendal nerve supplies the anus and perianal skin.

3 (a) **True** These ligaments are condensations of the visceral pelvic fascia and are the main supports of the uterus and upper vagina.
   (b) **False** The round ligament may prevent retroversion, but does not support the uterus.
   (c) **True** These condensations of fascia support the cervix.
   (d) **False** Unrepaired third-degree tear does not lead to uterine prolapse.
   (e) **False** This is a peritoneal fold and contains no supportive tissue.

4 (a) **True** Vaginal secretions come from the cervix and as an epithelial transudate.
   (b) **False** The glycogen is converted to lactic acid to keep the pH at around 4.5.
   (c) **True** The level at which the epithelium changes is known as the transformation zone.
   (d) **False** The portions are interstitial, isthmus, ampulla and fimbria from medial to lateral.
   (e) **False** The ovary is the only intra-abdominal structure that is not covered by peritoneum.

5 (a) **False** There is decreased fat deposition after the menopause.
   (b) **True** The presence of glycogen is oestrogen-dependent.
   (c) **False** The uterus atrophies after the menopause, and therefore the ratio increases.
   (d) **True**
   (e) **True** Due to maternal oestrogen effects. The pH increases after about 2 weeks.

NORMAL AND ABNORMAL SEXUAL DEVELOPMENT AND PUBERTY

6 Sexual differentiation:

   (a) Genetic sex is the same as gonadal sex
   (b) The presence of the second X-chromosome determines female differentiation
   (c) The Müllerian ducts develop into the internal organs of the female
   (d) The SRY gene on the Y-chromosome produces testicular determining factor
   (e) The 45XO phenotype is female

7 Puberty:

   (a) Puberty is preceded by decreasing pulses of follicle-stimulating hormone (FSH)
   (b) Breast development precedes the growth spurt
   (c) Pubic hair growth precedes axillary hair growth
   (d) Menarche occurs between 9 and 17 years of age
   (e) Menstrual cycles at menarche are usually regular

8 Patients with the following conditions typically present with primary amenorrhoea:

   (a) Uterus didelphys
   (b) Imperforate hymen
   (c) Anorexia nervosa
   (d) Testicular feminization
   (e) Untreated congenital adrenal hyperplasia

9 In Turner's syndrome:

   (a) A chromosomal structure of 45XY is characteristic
   (b) Secondary amenorrhoea is usual
   (c) Coarctation of the aorta may occur
   (d) The ovaries are multicystic
   (e) Pubic hair is absent

6 (a) **False** Embryo differentiation is genetic sex, while development of the gonad is gonadal sex.
   (b) **False** The lack of a Y-chromosome will result in the development of an ovary.
   (c) **True** The Wolffian duct develops into the male internal organs.
   (d) **True** This differentiates the gonad into a testis.
   (e) **True** As there is no Y-chromosome.

7 (a) **False** Increasing pulses of FSH precede puberty.
   (b) **False** The growth spurt occurs before breast development.
   (c) **True**
   (d) **True**
   (e) **False** The hypothalamic–pituitary axis may take several years to mature.

8 (a) **False** There is no effect on menstruation.
   (b) **True** Strictly speaking this causes cryptomenorrhoea (i.e. retention of menstrual secretion), but it is a differential diagnosis of primary amenorrhoea.
   (c) **False** This causes secondary amenorrhoea.
   (d) **True** The uterus is absent.
   (e) **True** Once treated with corticosteroids, normal menstruation occurs.

9 (a) **False** 45XO is the commonest karyotype. Mosaics such as XO, XX may also occur.
   (b) **False** There is primary amenorrhoea.
   (c) **True** It is well recognized as occurring in association with Turner's syndrome.
   (d) **False** The ovaries are streak-like structures.
   (e) **True** There is a lack of all secondary sexual characteristics.

10 Turner's syndrome:

(a) May not present until delayed puberty or infertility is diagnosed
(b) May have a male phenotype
(c) Is characterized by short stature, wide carrying angle and widely spaced nipples
(d) Is characterized by low oestrogen levels due to primary hypopituitarism
(e) The luteinizing hormone (LH) and FSH levels are usually markedly elevated

11 In testicular feminization:

(a) The chromosome status is XXY
(b) The gonads should be removed after puberty
(c) The patient adopts a male role and appearance
(d) Breasts are absent
(e) The voice is female

10 (a) **True** It may also be diagnosed soon after birth.
   (b) **False** Turner's syndrome (45XO) always has a female phenotype.
   (c) **True** Other features include colour blindness, coarctation and short metatarsals.
   (d) **False** Low oestrogen levels are due to ovarian failure.
   (e) **True** High LH and FSH levels are a response to gonadal failure.

11 (a) **False** The chromosome karyotype is XY.
   (b) **True** There is a 5% risk of development of dysgerminoma.
   (c) **False** They are invariably female in appearance.
   (d) **False** The breasts are fairly well developed after puberty.
   (e) **True** There is androgen insensitivity, so no masculinization of the larynx takes place.

THE NORMAL MENSTRUAL CYCLE

12 Menstruation:

    (a) Is not normally accompanied by pain
    (b) Involves the discharge of blood, mucus and the unfertilized ovum
    (c) The normal range of blood loss is 30–80 mL
    (d) Usually ceases before the age of 48 years
    (e) Is often followed by fluid retention

13 In the menstrual cycle, ovulation:

    (a) Occurs 2 days after the peak of LH
    (b) Occurs 14 days before the onset of the menstrual flow
    (c) Occurs when progesterone secretion is at maximal
    (d) Will only occur as a reflex response to orgasm
    (e) May be inhibited by emotional disturbance

14 Follicle-stimulating hormone (FSH):

    (a) Is responsible for oestradiol production from the granulosa cells
    (b) Brings about follicular rupture
    (c) Shows raised levels in polycystic ovary syndrome
    (d) Is necessary for the initial stages of follicle development
    (e) Is necessary for maintenance of the corpus luteum

12 (a) **False** Dysmenorrhoea may occur physiologically, especially in young and nulliparous women.
   (b) **False** The unfertilized ovum is autolyzed in the Fallopian tube several days prior to menstruation.
   (c) **True** There is wide variation, and a woman may find the loss excessive if it is an increase for her, even within this range.
   (d) **False** The median age at which the menopause occurs is 50 years.
   (e) **False** Fluid retention precedes menstruation.

13 (a) **False** Ovulation occurs about 36 hours after the onset of the LH surge (12 hours after the peak).
   (b) **True** The length of the luteal phase is fairly constant, unlike that of the follicular phase.
   (c) **False** Progesterone secretion increases very shortly before ovulation, reaching its peak in the mid-luteal phase.
   (d) **False** In some animals coitus stimulates ovulation, but not in humans.
   (e) **True** Pseudocyesis is a spectacular example.

14 (a) **True** The ovarian follicle (granulosa cells) is stimulated by FSH to produce oestradiol.
   (b) **False** LH is released mid-cycle, which brings about the changes which lead to oocyte release.
   (c) **False** LH levels are raised in this condition, relative to the FSH level.
   (d) **False** The very early stages of follicle development are hormone independent.
   (e) **False** LH promotes corpus luteum formation, and human chorionic gonadotrophin (HCG) stimulates its continuation.

DISORDERS OF THE MENSTRUAL CYCLE

15 Therapeutic indications for progestogens include:

(a) Endometriosis
(b) Fibroids
(c) Endometrial carcinoma
(d) Habitual abortion
(e) Dysfunctional uterine bleeding

16 The following are indications for oestrogen treatment:

(a) Fibroids
(b) Atrophic vulval dystrophy
(c) Postmenopausal vaginitis
(d) Threatened abortion
(e) Ovarian dysgenesis

17 The following investigations may be relevant in cases of amenorrhoea:

(a) Skull X-ray
(b) Pregnancy test
(c) Thyroid function tests
(d) Glucose tolerance test
(e) Gonadotrophin-releasing hormone (GnRH) estimation

18 In the polycystic ovary syndrome (PCOS):

(a) Obesity is common
(b) There is loss of body hair
(c) LH levels are low
(d) Irregular, widely spaced menstruation is typical
(e) Clomiphene may restore ovulation and menstruation

15 (a) **True** Continuous administration suppresses cyclical bleeding from the endometrium (both normal and ectopic).

(b) **False** Fibroids may enlarge if progestogens are given.

(c) **True** Regression of metastases and primary tumour occurs in a proportion of cases.

(d) **False** Although injections of progesterone have been widely used in the past for this purpose, there is no evidence of their efficacy.

(e) **True** It is particularly effective in cystic glandular hyperplasia.

16 (a) **False** Indeed, oestrogens may accelerate the growth of fibroids.

(b) **False** Although this condition appears after the menopause, it does not respond to oestrogen treatment. Hydrocortisone and testosterone creams are used symptomatically.

(c) **True** Oestrogen is effective when administered either orally or vaginally.

(d) **False** The use of synthetic oestrogens in pregnancy predisposes the exposed female fetus to cervical and vaginal neoplasia in later life.

(e) **True** Oestrogen will promote the development of breasts and secondary sexual characteristics in these patients.

17 (a) **True** This may be done to visualize the pituitary fossa.

(b) **True** One must never overlook the possibility of pregnancy.

(c) **True** Both myxoedema and hyperthyroidism may cause amenorrhoea.

(d) **False** Although severe diabetes may cause amenorrhoea, it is unlikely to be a presenting symptom.

(e) **False** GnRH stimulation tests are sometimes carried out, but GnRH assay is not routinely available.

18 (a) **True** When the condition was first described by Stein and Leventhal, obesity was thought to be invariably present. It is now recognized that not all women with PCO are obese.

(b) **False** There is usually hirsutism.

(c) **False** There is a relatively high LH level compared with FSH.

(d) **True** In the most extreme forms there is complete amenorrhoea, but oligomenorrhoea would be the most frequent pattern.

(e) **True** Clomiphene induces ovulation in about 70% of women with PCOS.

19 Postcoital bleeding may be a sign of:

    (a) Fibroids
    (b) Adenomatous polyps
    (c) Cervical ectropion
    (d) Dysplasia of the cervix
    (e) Carcinoma *in situ*

20 Heavy but regular periods are a likely feature of:

    (a) Fibroids
    (b) Carcinoma of the cervix
    (c) Dysfunctional uterine bleeding
    (d) Myxoedema
    (e) Hypertension

21 Cystic glandular hyperplasia:

    (a) Is associated with low oestrogen levels
    (b) May predispose to endometrial carcinoma
    (c) Is caused by a virus transmitted in cheese
    (d) Occurs with ovulatory failure
    (e) Generally occurs postmenopausally

22 Premenstrual tension syndrome:

    (a) Mostly occurs in women under 25 years
    (b) Is often accompanied by depression and irritability
    (c) Is only relieved when the menstrual flow is completed
    (d) Is exacerbated by psychosocial factors
    (e) May be associated with acts of crime

19 (a)   **True**   From a fibroid polyp.
   (b)   **True**   A benign endometrial polyp may, rarely, extrude through the cervix.
   (c)   **True**   The columnar epithelium of an ectropion is more likely to bleed slightly than squamous epithelium.
   (d and e) **False** The appearance of cervical dysplasia and carcinoma *in situ* to the naked eye is normal, and they do not cause symptoms.

20 (a) **True** Fibroids are a very common cause of menorrhagia.
   (b) **False** This usually causes irregular bleeding.
   (c) **True** The ovulatory forms of dysfunctional uterine bleeding are often regular. Anovulatory dysfunctional bleeding seen with severe polycystic ovary syndrome and at the extremes of reproductive life is irregular.
   (d) **True** In more severe cases of myxoedema, amenorrhoea may occur.
   (e) **False** Hypertension is not a cause of heavy periods.

21 (a) **False** In the early phase of the menopause, oestrogen levels are maintained but ovulation does not occur. This leads to a thickened cystic endometrium which sheds irregularly. Lack of progesterone means that the normal tortuosity and constrictor effect on spiral arterioles is lost.
   (b) **True** The endometrial hyperplasia may be atypical, with danger of progression to carcinoma.
   (c) **False** The histological appearance is sometimes described as being like 'Swiss cheese'. There the connection ends!
   (d) **True** The lack of ovulation and absence of progesterone lead to prolonged high levels of oestrogen.
   (e) **False** It occurs in puberty and perimenopausally.

22 (a) **False** It is commoner in women over 30 years.
   (b) **True** The cause of the emotional disturbance is not known.
   (c) **False** It is usually relieved by the *start* of the menstrual flow.
   (d) **True** In the management of the condition, recognition of adverse contributory factors is important.
   (e) **True** There is an increased incidence of shoplifting, etc., and even major acts of violence are said to occur more often in the premenstrual phase.

DISORDERS OF THE MENSTRUAL CYCLE

23 Effective treatments for primary dysmenorrhoea include:

(a) Diuretics
(b) Mefenamic acid
(c) Fenfluramine
(d) Combined contraceptive pills
(e) Presacral neurectomy

24 Abdominal hysterectomy has the following advantages over vaginal hysterectomy:

(a) It causes less postoperative pain
(b) The ovaries may be removed more easily if an unexpected endometrial cancer is discovered
(c) A large uterus is easily removed
(d) Prolapse can be repaired more adequately by plicating the uterosacral ligaments
(e) Postoperative recovery is more rapid

25 Dilatation and curettage (D & C):

(a) Should be carried out in all patients with menorrhagia
(b) Should be carried out in all patients with postmenopausal bleeding
(c) Should be recommended for all patients with breakthrough bleeding on oral contraception
(d) May be helpful in the diagnosis of ectopic pregnancy
(e) Is an essential investigation for subfertility

23 (a) **False** Diuretics may be helpful in the treatment of cyclical oedema, but not dysmenorrhoea.
   (b) **True** Prostaglandin inhibitors such as this may diminish uterine contractions.
   (c) **False** This agent is an appetite suppressant.
   (d) **True** Suppression of ovulation nearly always relieves dysmenorrhoea.
   (e) **True** This operation is not performed now, as there are simpler, effective treatments.

24 (a) **False** However, if posterior repair is carried out at the time of vaginal hysterectomy, considerable pain will be experienced.
   (b) **True** Some surgeons perform a dilatation and curettage (D & C) to exclude malignancy before vaginal hysterectomy.
   (c) **True** Removal of a large uterus vaginally often requires morcellation of the uterus.
   (d) **False** Vaginal hysterectomy with suture of the vault to the cardinal and uterosacral ligaments together with anterior and posterior repair (if required) is the standard operation.
   (e) **False** Many patients are ready to return home 2–3 days after vaginal hysterectomy.

25 (a) **False** If periods are heavy but still regular and the patient is less than, say, 35 years of age, an endometrial cancer is so unlikely that D & C is not mandatory.
   (b) **True** This applies even if another cause, such as atrophic vaginitis, is discovered. It is usually carried out with a hysterscopy now.
   (c) **False** However, it should be carried out if such bleeding persists after changing the oral contraceptive.
   (d) **True** Discovery of products of conception almost eliminates an ectopic pregnancy, while the presence of decidua with no trophoblast makes the diagnosis more likely.
   (e) **False** Ovulation can now be diagnosed biochemically, and a routine endometrial culture for tuberculosis is not essential in the UK.

FERTILITY CONTROL

26 The occlusive diaphragm:

(a) Should never be used for contraceptive purposes without contraceptive cream or jelly
(b) Has a similar Pearl index to the intrauterine contraceptive device (IUCD)
(c) Should be left *in situ* for at least 6 hours after intercourse
(d) Is less reliable than the cervical (Dumas) cap
(e) May be particularly beneficial for sex workers

27 The combined oral contraceptive:

(a) Predisposes to pelvic inflammatory disease
(b) Predisposes to benign breast disease and ovarian cysts
(c) Contains 0.2–0.5 mg of ethinyl oestradiol
(d) May be less effective in patients with epilepsy
(e) Works by causing an elevation in output of FSH and LH

28 Intrauterine contraceptive devices (IUCDs):

(a) Should not be inserted at the time of suction termination of pregnancy
(b) Are radio-opaque
(c) Should be removed in early pregnancy if the threads are visible
(d) Should preferably be inserted at mid-cycle
(e) Are contraindicated in patients with rheumatic heart disease

29 The following are absolute contraindications to use of the combined oral contraceptive:

(a) Varicose veins
(b) A previous history of viral hepatitis
(c) A prosthetic heart valve
(d) Diabetes mellitus
(e) Carcinoma *in situ* of the cervix

26 (a) **True** The diaphragm by itself has little contraceptive effect, and its function is to maintain a high concentration of spermicide at the cervical entrance.

   (b) **False** It is less reliable than the intrauterine device, having a Pearl index of 8–20, compared to less than 3 for the IUCD.

   (c) **True** If intercourse is to take place repeatedly within this time it should be left for 6 hours after the last intercourse.

   (d) **False** The failure rates are very similar.

   (e) **False** It does not protect against ascending infection or HIV transmission.

27 (a) **False**

   (b) **False** It protects against these conditions.

   (c) **False** It contains 20–50 µg (i.e. 0.02–0.05 mg).

   (d) **True** Hydantoins and barbiturates potentiate hepatic conjugation and excretion.

   (e) **False** It has multiple modes of action, but FSH and LH are suppressed.

28 (a) **False** There is no apparent increase in morbidity associated with this practice.

   (b) **True** It may be helpful to locate an IUCD on X-ray, although ultrasound is more usually used to locate a missing IUCD.

   (c) **True** The risk of an IUCD causing miscarriage is greater if it is left *in situ.*

   (d) **False** Shortly after menstruation is the recommended time.

   (e) **True** Insertion predisposes to bacterial endocarditis.

29 (a) **False** Thromboembolism is not more likely unless the veins themselves are part of the post-thrombotic leg.

   (b) **False** Provided that liver function has returned to normal it is quite safe to prescribe oral contraceptives.

   (c) **True** The added risk of thrombosis precludes the use of the oral contraceptive.

   (d) **False** Insulin requirements may increase slightly, but this is not an absolute contraindication.

   (e) **False** The oral contraceptive is not carcinogenic with regard to the cervix.

30 The following conditions are aggravated by the combined oral contraceptive:

(a) Hirsutism
(b) Endometriosis
(c) Dysmenorrhoea
(d) Premenstrual tension
(e) Cervical ectropion

31 The risks of use of the intrauterine device in nulliparous women include:

(a) Sterility
(b) Elevated serum copper levels
(c) Endometrial cancer
(d) Ectopic pregnancy
(e) Dyspareunia

32 Depo-Provera:

(a) Is usually used when contraception is required for more than 2 years
(b) Causes amenorrhoea in more than 50% of cases
(c) Does not prevent conception after 4 months
(d) Should be given every 3 months
(e) Prevents endometrial hyperplasia

33 Laparoscopic clip sterilization:

(a) Can be reversed with greater success than vasectomy
(b) May be surgically reversed with better results than for postinfective tubal occlusion
(c) Is associated with a failure rate of 1–2 in 1000
(d) Has a higher failure rate when performed at the time of termination of pregnancy
(e) Always requires general anaesthesia

30 (a) **False** Suppression of gonadotrophins decreases ovarian androgen production and this, together with the direct effect of oestrogen, may slightly improve hirsutism.
   (b) **False** Oestrogens by themselves aggravate endometriosis, but the combined pill causes shrinkage of normal and ectopic endometrium.
   (c) **False** Elimination of ovulation usually improves these symptoms.
   (d) **False**
   (e) **True** Cervical ectropion commonly occurs in women who have been on the pill.

31 (a) **True** This is because of ascending infection giving rise to salpingitis, which may be silent.
   (b) **False** The quantity of copper ions released is minute and does not affect serum levels.
   (c) **False** Although endometritis and increased menstrual loss may occur, there is no evidence to suggest that endometrial cancer is a risk.
   (d) **True** The risk is greater than with barrier methods or ovulation inhibitors, but the risk per cycle is not increased compared with that for women using no contraception.
   (e) **True** Dyspareunia probably occurs in relation to mild infection.

32 (a) **False** It is licensed for short-term use, although many consider it safe for longer-term use.
   (b) **True** Its effectiveness lasts for at least 3 months.
   (c) **False** Its duration of action is variable after 3 months.
   (d) **True** Although the duration of action may be as long as 6 months, 3 months is the maximal period on which one can rely.
   (e) **True** Like other progestogens, it suppresses endometrium.

33 (a) **True** Antisperm antibodies reduce the success of vasectomy reversal.
   (b) **True** Around 80% patency and 50% pregnancy rates can be expected after microscopic reanastomosis, and even better results have been reported from selected centres. The outlook for surgical repair after tubal diathermy is very poor.
   (c) **True** Couples should be warned of this.
   (d) **True** The increased vascularity if the woman is or has recently been pregnant increases the risk of recanalization.
   (e) **False** Local anaesthesia can be used.

FERTILITY CONTROL

34 Termination of pregnancy:

(a) May legally be performed at any gestation when there are severe fetal abnormalities
(b) Can be performed using prostaglandins
(c) Must be approved by three independent medical practitioners
(d) May be performed using Mifepristone (RU 486) up to 12 weeks' gestation
(e) Can be safely performed by suction before 14 weeks' gestation

35 Mid-trimester abortion with prostaglandins:

(a) Is illegal after 20 weeks' gestation
(b) May result in uterine rupture
(c) May cause cervical laceration
(d) May cause convulsions
(e) Usually takes more than 24 hours

36 In the UK, termination of pregnancy requires:

(a) Consent from the partner as well as the woman
(b) A surgical operation
(c) Consent from the guardian of a minor
(d) The agreement of any two doctors
(e) Notification of the Department of Health

37 Pregnancy may be terminated using:

(a) Prostaglandin inhibitors
(b) Progesterone inhibitors
(c) Suction evacuation
(d) Hygroscopic (hydrophilic) plastic dilators
(e) Beta-agonists

34 (a) **True** The 1992 changes to the abortion law allow termination for fetal abnormalities at any gestation, but restrict termination for other indications to below 24 weeks.

(b) **True** Prostaglandins can be administered by pessary or extra-amniotic injection.

(c) **False** Two practitioners must certify that there are legal grounds for termination.

(d) **False** Mifepristone must be used in conjunction with a vaginal prostaglandin or oral Misoprostol, and is only licensed for use prior to 9 weeks' gestation.

(e) **True** This is the most widely used method for first-trimester termination.

35 (a) **False** The upper limit of gestation is 24 weeks, and in cases of gross fetal abnormality the pregnancy may be terminated at any stage.

(b) **False** The uterus does not rupture as a result of termination.

(c) **True** Unduly strong contractions may cause cervical laceration.

(d) **False** Excessive use of oxytocin may cause water intoxication and convulsions, but not with the use of prostaglandins alone.

(e) **False** Abortion is usually complete within 12–24 hours.

36 (a) **False** Only the woman's consent is required.

(b) **False** Prostaglandins and anti-progesterones are just two of the pharmaceutical agents which may be used for termination.

(c) **False** If the girl is under 16 years of age, the parents should be consulted, but only if the doctor thinks it is in the girl's best interest.

(d) **False** Only *registered* medical practitioners who are not in partnership may sign the certificate (except in an emergency procedure when only one signature is required).

(e) **True** The doctor who terminates the pregnancy has an obligation to fill in the prescribed notification form and send it to the Department of Health.

37 (a) **False** It is prostaglandins themselves which may be used.

(b) **True** Mifepristone, an anti-progesterone, may be used in conjunction with prostaglandin.

(c) **True** This method can be used up to 13–14 weeks, or even later by a skilled operator.

(d) **False** These are used for cervical preparation and do not result in termination of pregnancy when used in isolation.

(e) **False** These relax uterine contractions in later pregnancy.

INFERTILITY

38 Bromocriptine:

(a) Is an analogue of prolactin
(b) Is used to treat hyperprolactinaemia
(c) Is a potent cause of multiple pregnancy
(d) May cause hypotension
(e) Effectively inhibits lactation after delivery

39 Gonadotrophin-releasing hormone (GnRH):

(a) Stimulates the release of FSH as well as LH
(b) Is a peptide of high molecular weight
(c) May be administered by single injection to stimulate ovulation
(d) When given in high dosage causes pituitary desensitization and a fall in FSH and LH
(e) Is produced by acidophilic cells of the anterior pituitary

40 The following values of a semen analysis indicate *abnormal* semen quality:

(a) Volume of less than 2 mL
(b) Density of 40 million/mL
(c) Motility of 40%
(d) Abnormal forms with an incidence of 40%
(e) Liquefaction complete in 30 minutes

41 Gonadotrophin-releasing hormone (GnRH) agonists:

(a) Must be given by pump
(b) Cause initial gonadotrophin release
(c) Are effective in the treatment of endometriosis
(d) Cause bone loss
(e) Relieve menopausal hot flushes

42 The following are acceptable methods for confirmation of ovulation:

(a) A drop in basal body temperature of at least 0.5°C on day 14
(b) A blood progesterone level on day 21
(c) Histological examination of premenstrual endometrial biopsy
(d) Blood oestrogen level on day 13
(e) Demonstration of spinnbarkeit in cervical mucus

38 (a) **False** It is a derivative of ergot alkaloid.
   (b) **True** It has an inhibitory effect on pituitary cells, so less prolactin is produced.
   (c) **False** It is not associated with multiple ovulation.
   (d) **True** This is less likely to occur if the dosage is increased slowly and the tablet is given at night.
   (e) **True** However, rebound lactation may occur if it is stopped abruptly.

39 (a) **True** It is secreted in a pulsatile fashion and stimulates the release of FSH and LH.
   (b) **False** It is a low-molecular-weight decapeptide.
   (c) **False** Its activity depends on pulsatility. Continuous administration diminishes gondatotrophin secretion by down-regulating its own receptor.
   (d) **True** This blocking action is utilized with the synthetic GnRH analogues to render women amenorrhoeic.
   (e) **False** It is produced by neurosecretory cells in the hypothalamus.

40 (a) **True** The normal volume is 2–5 mL.
   (b) **False** A count of below 20 million/mL justifies a diagnosis of oligospermia.
   (c) **True** Motility should be at least 50%.
   (d) **False** More than 70% of sperm need to be abnormal forms to indicate likely subfertility on account of morphology.
   (e) **False** This is the normal liquefaction time.

41 (a) **False** GnRH itself is given by pump. The analogue (agonist) is given by nasal spray or injection.
   (b) **True** They are *agonists*. Commercially available antagonists are under development.
   (c) **True** With continued use they down-regulate the pituitary. Endometriosis will usually recur when treatment is stopped.
   (d) **True** Due to hypo-oestrogenism.
   (e) **False** Flushes are a side-effect.

42 (a) **False** A rise in temperature of 0.5°C must be maintained over the last 14 days of the cycle.
   (b) **True** Progesterone reaches a mid-luteal peak.
   (c) **True** Secretory changes in the endometrium only occur after ovulation.
   (d) **False** Oestrogen levels indicate follicular development but not ovulation.
   (e) **False** This is a pre-ovulatory phenomenon that is dependent on oestrogen.

43 Tubal patency may properly be demonstrated by:

(a) Hysterosalpingography
(b) Air insufflation
(c) Laparoscopy and methylene-blue dye insufflation
(d) Computerized tomography (CT) scan
(e) Hysteroscopy

44 The following are recognized complications of treatment of anovulatory infertility:

(a) Multiple pregnancy
(b) Ectopic pregnancy
(c) Cervical mucus hostility
(d) Postural hypotension
(e) Ascites

45 Clomiphene citrate:

(a) Results in decreased cervical mucus production
(b) Blocks FSH release
(c) Results in increased GnRH release
(d) Directly stimulates follicular growth
(e) May result in ovarian hyperstimulation

46 In male factor infertility:

(a) Men with hypogonadotrophic hypogonadism respond to mesterolone (testosterone analogue)
(b) Tamoxifen may increase spermatogenesis
(c) Steroids may decrease antisperm antibody levels
(d) The postcoital test is usually positive
(e) May be helped by intracytoplasmic sperm injection (ICSI)

43 (a) **True** Injection of a radio-opaque dye is usually screened on an image intensifier prior to taking X-ray pictures.

   (b) **False** Insufflation with carbon dioxide is acceptable, but with air there is a grave risk of air embolus.

   (c) **True** In many centres this is now the method of choice for assessing tubal patency.

   (d) **False** CT is not helpful for this procedure.

   (e) **False** Hysteroscopy examines the uterine cavity, not the tubes.

44 (a) **True** Both clomiphene and gonadotrophin therapy may cause multiple ovulation and hence multiple pregnancy.

   (b) **False** Tubal surgery and *in vitro* fertilization may result in ectopic pregnancy, but not ovulatory stimulation *per se*.

   (c) **True** Clomiphene (anti-oestrogenic effect) may render cervical mucus hostile.

   (d) **True** This is a classical side-effect when bromocriptine treatment is started.

   (e) **True** Gonadotrophin hyperstimulation leads to ovarian cyst formation and ascites.

45 (a) **True** The anti-oestrogenic effect of clomiphene may render cervical mucus thick.

   (b) **False** It is an anti-oestrogen which increases gonadotrophin production.

   (c) **True** It blocks the oestrogen-receptor sites in the hypothalamus, and so stimulates increased GnRH release.

   (d) **False** Its actions are mediated by restoration of FSH secretion.

   (e) **True** The full-blown clinical syndrome is very rare with clomiphene used by itself.

46 (a) **False** Gonadotrophins are necessary.

   (b) **True** However, the fertility rate is not improved.

   (c) **True** An increase in fertility is also reported with relatively high doses of steroids.

   (d) **False** A negative postcoital test is quite often the first pointer to male factor infertility.

   (e) **True** Intracytoplasmic injection allows fertilization of oocytes with low sperm densities.

47 During a vaginal examination, the diagnosis of vaginismus is
   suggested by:

   (a) Profuse vaginal discharge
   (b) Involuntary spasm of levator ani muscles
   (c) Involuntary abduction of the hips
   (d) Congenital vaginal stenosis
   (e) Imperforate hymen

48 Orgasmic dysfunction in women can be due to:

   (a) Neurological problems
   (b) Vaginismus
   (c) Inadequate clitoral stimulation
   (d) Fear of losing control
   (e) Pregnancy

47 (a) **False** Vaginismus is an involuntary spasm of the levator ani due to fear.
  (b) **True** It is usually fear of pain that causes the spasm.
  (c) **False** It is the adduction of the hips that prevents examination.
  (d) **False** Mechanical vaginal obstruction does not cause vaginismus.
  (e) **False**

48 (a) **True** Long-standing diabetes and multiple sclerosis are recognized causes of sexual disorders.
  (b) **False** Women with vaginismus are usually orgasmic with clitoral stimulation.
  (c) **True** This is the commonest cause of anorgasmia.
  (d) **True**
  (e) **False** Some women may fear that orgasm will be harmful to the pregnancy, but there is no evidence to that effect.

DISORDERS OF EARLY PREGNANCY

49 In threatened abortion:

(a) The uterine size is typically less than expected for the period of gestation
(b) Progesterone therapy is useful
(c) Pain is absent
(d) Vaginal bleeding is present in most cases
(e) Bed rest may prevent miscarriage

50 Causes of first-trimester abortion include:

(a) Malaria infection
(b) Rubella
(c) Syphilis
(d) XO karyotype in the embryo
(e) Trisomy 21 in the embryo

51 Septic abortion:

(a) May result from exposure to gonorrhoea during pregnancy
(b) Is frequently due to a combination of coliforms and bacteroides
(c) Is more likely to lead to septic shock than salpingitis or pelvic abscess in a non-pregnant patient
(d) Should be treated by immediate curettage of the uterus in all cases
(e) Is a less common cause of maternal death in the UK than it was 20 years ago

49 (a) **False** This is a feature of missed abortion.
   (b) **False** Progesterone has been shown not to help, and it may interfere with external genital development in continuing pregnancies.
   (c) **True** By definition, a threatened abortion is bleeding in early pregnancy without pain.
   (d) **False** By definition, vaginal bleeding is *always* present.
   (e) **False** Bed rest has been shown to confer no benefit.

50 (a) **True** Any high fever can cause abortion, but malaria is particularly likely to do so because *Plasmodium* parasitizes the chorio-decidual space.
   (b) **True** Although the association between rubella and congenital defects is better known, acute rubella may result in miscarriage.
   (c) **False** The spirochaete does not cross the placenta until after 20 weeks of pregnancy.
   (d) **True** This is the commonest chromosomal abnormality in abortion material.
   (e) **True** Around 80% of 'Down's' embryos are aborted.

51 (a) **False** The cervical plug is a very effective barrier to ascending infection during pregnancy.
   (b) **True** Since these organisms are commonly present in the vagina and perineum, they often infect an incomplete abortion.
   (c) **True** Pregnant patients are particularly predisposed to endotoxic shock.
   (d) **False** (i) Where bleeding is not heavy and the patient has a very high temperature, curettage should be deferred for 6–12 hours to give time for antibiotics to take effect. Immediate surgical interference may lead to septic shock. However, any pieces of infective material in the cervix should be removed with sponge forceps.
      (ii) If the uterus is over 14 weeks in size, contractions should be induced by an oxytocin infusion.
   (e) **True** This is due at least in part to the introduction of legal abortion.

52 In the diagnosis of ectopic pregnancy:

(a) A ruptured corpus luteum cyst may cause identical clinical features
(b) Vaginal bleeding will be present in 99% of all cases
(c) The standard urinary pregnancy test is very useful
(d) Pain usually precedes vaginal bleeding
(e) A history of 10 weeks of amenorrhoea and pain in a patient who usually has 28-day cycles is highly suggestive

53 Ectopic pregnancy:

(a) Is associated with uterine enlargement
(b) Is situated in the ovary in about 0.5% of all cases
(c) Is more dangerous when it is situated in the isthmus of the Fallopian tube
(d) Can only be diagnosed after it has ruptured
(e) Is a complication of assisted conception

54 Cervical incompetence:

(a) Typically causes painful abortions
(b) Typically causes mid-trimester abortion
(c) Is treated by cervical cerclage which is best performed early in the second trimester
(d) May be caused by hydramnios
(e) May lead to premature rupture of the membranes

55 In ectopic pregnancy:

(a) Bleeding precedes pain
(b) Shoulder-tip pain is an important symptom
(c) The isthmus of the tube is the commonest site of implantation
(d) The incidence is higher in women fitted with intrauterine devices
(e) Ultrasonic scan is of no help in diagnosis

52 (a) **True** This causes intraperitoneal haemorrhage (which is often considerable) after a short period of amenorrhoea. The differential diagnosis is difficult, and may only be clarified by laparoscopy.
   (b) **False** It is present in about 85% of cases. It is often absent in those acute ectopics with intraperitoneal rupture of the isthmus.
   (c) **False** It is invariably positive, but the quantitative serum βhCG test may be useful.
   (d) **True** Pain usually comes first, in contrast to spontaneous abortion.
   (e) **False** Patients with ectopic pregnancy usually have a short history of amenorrhoea, 6–8 weeks from the start of the last period; 10 weeks would suggest inevitable abortion.

53 (a) **True** Although uterine enlargement occurs under the influence of oestrogen and progesterone, it is not as large as an intrauterine pregnancy.
   (b) **True** Ovarian implantation is a rare site for ectopic pregnancy.
   (c) **True** This tends to lead to tubal rupture and massive intraperitoneal haemorrhage. Ampullary implantation more often leads to 'tubal abortion' with a more gradual accumulation of blood.
   (d) **False** The increasing use of sensitive βhCG tests and transvaginal ultrasound often allows diagnosis of ectopic pregnancy prior to rupture.
   (e) **True** There is a threefold increase in incidence with *in vitro* fertilization (IVF) and gamete intrafallopian transfer (GIFT).

54 (a) **False** The 'incompetent' cervix dilates easily; thus abortion is relatively pain-free in typical cases.
   (b) **True** It is doubtful whether it is ever a cause of first-trimester loss.
   (c) **True** First-trimester abortion for other reasons is common (15–20% of all pregnancies); therefore, cerclage is best delayed until the second trimester.
   (d) **False** Hydramnios leads to premature delivery in its own right.
   (e) **True** The incompetent cervix typically presents with painless dilatation, followed by rupture of the membranes.

55 (a) **False** Pain usually precedes bleeding.
   (b) **True** Blood tracks up the paracolic gutters to the diaphragm, where it causes referred pain.
   (c) **False** The ampulla is the commonest site.
   (d) **True** The copper-containing devices probably interfere with tubal motility and ciliary function.
   (e) **False** Tubal pregnancy is often identified on transvaginal ultrasonic scan, and the scan is also helpful for excluding an intrauterine pregnancy when the βhCG test is positive.

DISORDERS OF EARLY PREGNANCY

56 Complications of hydatidiform mole include:

(a) Hyperemesis gravidarum
(b) Malignant change
(c) Haemorrhage
(d) Diabetes insipidus
(e) Development of ovarian cysts

57 First-trimester abortion may be due to:

(a) Inadequate oestrogen production
(b) Chromosomal abnormality of the fetus
(c) Incompetence of the internal cervical os
(d) Maternal diabetes
(e) Cytotoxic drugs

56 (a) **True** This is thought to be due to the excessive production of chorionic gondadotrophin.
   (b) **True** Around 2–10% progress to choriocarcinoma, the incidence varying in different parts of the world.
   (c) **True** Expulsion of the mole or surgical evacuation may be associated with haemorrhage.
   (d) **False** There is no association with diabetes insipidus (or mellitus).
   (e) **True** Theca lutein cysts of the ovary may develop due to stimulation by chorionic gonadotrophin.

57 (a) **False** This theory has been discredited.
   (b) **True** Around 60% of abortion material has been found to be chromosomally abnormal.
   (c) **False** Cervical incompetence causes mid-trimester abortion.
   (d) **True** Poorly controlled diabetes may cause abortion.
   (e) **True** For this reason, cytotoxic drugs would not knowingly be given in pregnancy.

BENIGN DISEASE OF THE UTERUS AND CERVIX

58 The following organisms are known causes of pelvic inflammatory disease:

(a) *Streptococcus pyogenes*
(b) *Herpes simplex*
(c) *Chlamydia*
(d) *Clostridium welchii*
(e) *Trichomonas*

59 Tuberculosis of the female genital tract:

(a) Most commonly affects the Fallopian tubes
(b) Is usually sexually transmitted
(c) May cause ascites
(d) Causes infertility
(e) Is best diagnosed by taking an endometrial biopsy in the first half of the cycle

60 In women with syphilis:

(a) The incubation period may be as long as 3 months
(b) A chancre will be seen in most cases
(c) If the venereal disease research laboratory (VDRL) slide test is positive, the *Treponema pallidum* haemagglutination (TPHA) will be negative
(d) General paralysis of the insane may result
(e) Tetracyclines may be used for treatment

61 Chlamydial infection is:

(a) The most common cause of sexually transmitted diseases (STD)
(b) Caused by an intracellular organism
(c) Silent in over 50% of cases
(d) Sensitive to metronidazole
(e) A possible cause of pneumonia in infants

58 (a) **True** This organism is often responsible for post-abortion or post-delivery infection.
  (b) **False** *Herpes simplex* infection is confined to the vagina and cervix.
  (c) **True** This and *Neiserria gonococci* cause more than two-thirds of cases, but super-infection with other organisms usually occurs.
  (d) **True** Infection may occur following criminal abortion.
  (e) **False** This organism only affects the vagina.

59 (a) **True** The tubes and endometrium are invariably affected.
  (b) **False** It is nearly always secondary to pulmonary tuberculosis.
  (c) **True** This is now a rare cause of ascites in the UK.
  (d) **True** The tubes are almost invariably infected and, even after full chemotherapy, restoration of fertility is unusual.
  (e) **False** It is necessary to take a biopsy in the second half of the cycle when the granulomata have had time to develop.

60 (a) **True** The incubation period may be from 9 to 90 days.
  (b) **False** Women usually present with secondary disease because the chancre is not noticed as it is not exposed.
  (c) **False** The VDRL is based on IgM and becomes negative more rapidly than the TPHA after successful treatment.
  (d) **True** This is fortunately now a rare manifestation of neurosyphilis.
  (e) **True** This is second-line treatment for patients allergic to penicillin.

61 (a) **True** Infection due to *Chlamydia* is now the most common sexually transmitted disease.
  (b) **True** It is a Gram-negative intracellular obligate bacterium.
  (c) **True** It is commonly harboured in the cervix without symptoms.
  (d) **False** It is sensitive to tetracycline and erythromycin.
  (e) **True** The more common neonatal infection is ophthalmia neonatorum.

62 Human immunodeficiency virus (HIV) carriers:

(a) Are always serum antibody positive
(b) Have a better prognosis with treatment
(c) Cannot transmit the disease until they develop the clinical syndrome
(d) Transmit the virus to the fetus in over 80% of cases
(e) Will almost certainly not develop the disease

63 Gonorrhoea:

(a) Infects the vaginal epithelium
(b) May cause arthritis
(c) May be symptomless
(d) Is diagnosed by a serological test
(e) Crosses the placenta

64 Tubal damage is a recognized complication of:

(a) Asymptomatic chlamydial salpingitis
(b) Pneumococcal salpingitis
(c) Intrauterine devices
(d) Ovarian cystectomy
(e) Actinomycosis

65 Acceptable treatment for uterine fibroids includes:

(a) No treatment
(b) Myomectomy during pregnancy if red degeneration occurs
(c) Cyclical oestrogen treatment
(d) Vaginal myomectomy
(e) Caesarean hysterectomy

66 Fibroids:

(a) May protrude through the cervix
(b) Are composed mainly of fibrous tissue
(c) Are more common in infertile patients
(d) Are rare in Afro-Caribbean women
(e) Commonly arise from the cervix

62 (a) **False** Most cases develop antibodies within 3 months of infection.
(b) **True** Many of the opportunistic infections may be prevented or improved with appropriate antibiotics, and antiviral agents may slow the progression.
(c) **False** An HIV-positive patient is just as potentially infective as someone with AIDS.
(d) **False** Transplacental spread occurs in less than 50% of cases.
(e) **False** At the present time, virtually all HIV-positive patients will eventually progress to AIDS.

63 (a) **False** It infects glandular epithelium such as that of the cervix or urethra.
(b) **True** Bloodborne spread to joints, endocardium and iris is rare.
(c) **True** In women, symptoms are often mild or non-existent.
(d) **False** The gonoccocal complement fixation test is unreliable and does not become positive until several weeks after infection.
(e) **False** Gonoccocal ophthalmia may be acquired by the baby during delivery, but the organism does not cross the placenta.

64 (a) **True** Ascending infection can occur, resulting in tubal damage without any symptoms.
(b) **False**
(c) **True** Ascending pelvic infections are more common, especially in nulliparous women.
(d) **True** The fimbriae may become involved in peritubal adhesions.
(e) **True** This is a well-recognized infection in association with intrauterine devices.

65 (a) **True** If tumours are small (less than the size of a 12-week pregnancy) and asymptomatic, this is the appropriate management.
(b) **False** This can be highly dangerous, causing severe haemorrhage, and is likely to initiate labour.
(c) **False** This tends to cause enlargement of fibroids.
(d) **True** This is appropriate for pedunculated submucous fibroids.
(e) **True** If no further pregnancies are desired.

66 (a) **True** Submucosal fibroids may become polypoid and be extruded through the cervix where they ulcerate and become infected.
(b) **False** They are composed mainly of smooth muscle.
(c) **True** They are more common in people who are subfertile and, once formed, they may contribute further to subfertility.
(d) **False** They are three times more common in Afro-Caribbean than in Caucasian women.
(e) **False** Only 2% of fibroids arise from this site.

BENIGN DISEASE OF THE UTERUS AND CERVIX

67 Complications of fibroids include:

(a) Intraperitoneal haemorrhage
(b) Endometrial carcinoma
(c) Obstructed labour
(d) Polycythaemia
(e) Recurrent abortion

67 (a) **True** From rupture of a surface vessel.
   (b) **False** Sarcoma is found in 0.2% of cases.
   (c) **True** A pelvic fibroid may obstruct labour.
   (d) **True** This is probably due to erythropoietin secretion by the tumour.
   (e) **True** Submucous fibroids in particular may interfere with implantation and cause abortion.

BENIGN DISEASE OF THE UTERUS AND CERVIX

ENDOMETRIOSIS

68 Endometriosis is a recognized cause of:

(a) Deep dyspareunia
(b) Amenorrhoea
(c) Dysmenorrhoea
(d) Postmenopausal bleeding
(e) Painful laparotomy scar

69 Endometriosis:

(a) Is the commonest cause of chronic lower abdominal pain in young women
(b) Most frequently involves the ovaries
(c) Often flares up during pregnancy
(d) Is associated with subfertility
(e) Is more common in Afro-Caribbean women

70 The following are useful for the treatment of endometriosis:

(a) Danazol
(b) Dydrogesterone
(c) GnRH analogues
(d) The oral contraceptive
(e) Prednisolone

71 Chronic pelvic pain:

(a) May be a manifestation of underlying psychological distress
(b) Should always be investigated by laparotomy
(c) Is by definition cyclical
(d) Is a frequent symptom of chronic pelvic inflammatory disease
(e) Is most common in postmenopausal women

72 Low backache in women is associated with:

(a) A retroverted uterus
(b) Premenstrual syndrome
(c) Gynaecological abnormalities more often than musculoskeletal problems
(d) Long-standing endometriosis
(e) Pregnancy

68 (a) **True** This is one of the classical features, together with dysmenorrhoea, pain and menorrhagia.
   (b) **False** Significant hormone imbalance is not a feature.
   (c) **True** Cyclical bleeding into or from the deposits causes pain prior to and during menstruation.
   (d) **False** Endometriotic deposits usually regress after the menopause.
   (e) **True** Rarely, ectopic endometrium may appear in scars.

69 (a) **False** In most cases of chronic pelvic pain, no cause is found.
   (b) **True** The peritoneum of the broad ligament and pouch of Douglas are the next commonest site.
   (c) **False** The disease regresses during pregnancy.
   (d) **True** The mechanism involved is not clearly understood, as ovulation and tubal patency are usually maintained.
   (e) **False** Fibroids are more common in Afro-Caribbeans; endometriosis is more common in Caucasians.

70 (a) **True** Danazol, a weak androgen with anti-oestrogenic action, suppresses menstruation but may have severe side-effects.
   (b) **True** Synthetic progestogen also suppresses menstruation if given continuously. Side-effects include weight gain and fluid retention.
   (c) **True** These act by suppressing pituitary gonadotrophin production, and amenorrhoea results.
   (d) **True** The beneficial effect is due to the progestogen.
   (e) **False** Corticosteroids have no effect on endometriosis.

71 (a) **True** However, psychogenic pain should not be diagnosed until organic causes have been excluded.
   (b) **False** Ultrasound and laparoscopy are the two most useful investigations.
   (c) **False** Dysmenorrhoea, mittelschmerz and pelvic congestion are examples of cyclical pain. Other causes are often non-cyclical.
   (d) **True** Although the severity of pain is variable, it is the cardinal symptom of pelvic inflammatory disease.
   (e) **False** Both organic and psychogenic causes of pelvic pain are unusual after the menopause.

72 (a) **False** Uncomplicated retroversion, without fixation, does not cause backache.
   (b) **True** There is often premenstrual low back pain.
   (c) **False** Backache is far more likely to be due to lumbo-sacral injuries/abnormalities.
   (d) **True** When endometriosis involves the utero-sacral ligaments, with fixed retroversion, there is often chronic low back pain.
   (e) **True** Pregnancy often exacerbates or unmasks a lumbo-sacral cause of back pain.

BENIGN DISEASE OF THE OVARY

73 Physiological follicular cysts:

(a) Are the commonest benign ovarian tumours
(b) Result from the non-rupture of the corpus luteum
(c) Never persist after the end of the menstrual cycle
(d) Rarely reach a diameter of 10 cm
(e) Require intervention if they become symptomatic

74 Dermoid cysts:

(a) Are germ-cell tumours
(b) Are usually bilateral
(c) Are the commonest cysts detected during pregnancy
(d) Are commonly malignant
(e) Are frequently 46XY in chromosome complement

75 Epithelial cell tumours:

(a) Mucinous cystadenoma is the commonest variety
(b) They occur mainly in women over 40 years of age
(c) Cystadenomas of the mucinous variety are the largest
(d) Endometroid cystadenoma is the same as ovarian endometriosis
(e) Brenner tumours may turn malignant

BENIGN DISEASE OF THE OVARY

73 (a) **True**
   (b) **False** They result from the non-rupture/atresia of the dominant follicle.
   (c) **False** They may persist for several menstrual cycles.
   (d) **True** They usually do not exceed 5–6 cms in diameter.
   (e) **True** Symptoms due to haemorrhage or torsion may require surgical intervention.

74 (a) **True** They are germ-cell tumours or teratomas.
   (b) **False** They are bilateral in 10–12% of cases.
   (c) **True** They are the commonest cysts detected during pregnancy.
   (d) **False** They are malignant in less than 5% of cases.
   (e) **False** They are always 46XX.

75 (a) **False** Serous cystadenoma is the commonest variety.
   (b) **True** Malignant cysts occur in the older age group.
   (c) **True** They are typically extremely large.
   (d) **False** Although they are difficult to differentiate macroscopically, they are histologically different and have different aetiologies.
   (e) **True** Rarely they may become malignant.

MALIGNANT DISEASE OF THE UTERUS AND CERVIX

76 Cervical smears:

    (a) Are taken with a throat swab
    (b) Should be placed in fixative immediately
    (c) Should be taken every 10 years
    (d) Should be followed by colposcopy if any abnormality is reported
    (e) Should not be taken in women under 21 years of age

77 Carcinoma *in situ* of the cervix:

    (a) Arises from the squamo-columnar junction
    (b) Usually becomes invasive within 3–4 years
    (c) Causes a mosaic appearance on colposcopy
    (d) May regress spontaneously
    (e) Merges gradually with healthy epithelium

78 Cone biopsy of the cervix:

    (a) Should be performed on all patients with carcinoma *in situ* unless hysterectomy is required for some other reason
    (b) May cause secondary haemorrhage, with a peak incidence 14–21 days after the operation
    (c) Has been performed more frequently since the discovery of colposcopy
    (d) Is required for symptomatic cervical erosions
    (e) Increases the likelihood of Caesarean section in a subsequent pregnancy

79 Endocervical carcinoma:

    (a) Is usually an adenocarcinoma
    (b) May spread directly to para-aortic nodes
    (c) Usually causes death from local invasion before metastases become manifest
    (d) Causes a barrel-shaped cervix
    (e) Is usually diagnosed by means of a cone biopsy

76 (a) **False** An Ayre's spatula (or variant) or a cervical brush is used.
   (b) **True** Air drying spoils the preparation.
   (c) **False** Ideally a smear should be repeated every 3 years.
   (d) **False** All cases of cervical intra-epithelial neoplasia (CIN) should be referred for colposcopy. If the smear only reports inflammatory changes, it should be repeated after treatment.
   (e) **False** All sexually active women should have smears taken regularly.

77 (a) **True**
   (b) **False** Ten years is the mean time for invasive change.
   (c) **True** This appearance is caused by abnormal capillary patterns.
   (d) **True** The exact proportion of CIN cases which will spontaneously regress is not known, but it is certainly considerable.
   (e) **False** The junction between healthy and abnormal epithelium is abrupt.

78 (a) **False** Laser treatment, coagulation or some other form of 'ablation' may be employed, provided that the whole ectocervix can be inspected through the colposcope.
   (b) **False** The peak incidence for secondary haemorrhage is 7–10 days postoperatively.
   (c) **False** Colposcopy allows selective biopsy of the affected areas to be performed, and ablation if no invasion is detected. Cone biopsy can therefore be reserved for those cases where the squamo-columnar junction is high in the endocervical canal and cannot be visualized through the colposcope.
   (d) **False** These are treated by cryosurgery or coagulation.
   (e) **True** Cervical stenosis (fibrosis) may prevent dilatation, although no difficulty is experienced in the majority of cases.

79 (a) **False** Squamous metaplasia usually precedes malignancy.
   (b) **True** In this case, spread occurs along the ovarian lymphatics.
   (c) **True** As with ectocervical cancer, renal failure (due to ureteric obstruction) is the commonest cause of death.
   (d) **True**
   (e) **False** This is used for carcinoma *in situ* and dysplasia when an adequate colposcopically directed biopsy is impossible, most often because the squamo-columnar junction cannot be seen.

80 Stage I cancer of the cervix:

(a) Is confined to the uterus
(b) May not be visible on clinical examination
(c) Has a better prognosis than stage I cancer of the endometrium
(d) May be associated with hydro-ureter on intravenous pyelogram
(e) May be treated with intracavity radiation (to provide 7000 rads at point A) and external radiotherapy

81 Radiotherapy for carcinoma of the cervix may cause:

(a) Vesico-vaginal fistula
(b) Pyometra
(c) Proctitis
(d) Acute salpingitis
(e) Ovarian failure

82 Carcinoma of the endometrium:

(a) Is very rare (incidence of less than 5%) before the menopause
(b) Is more common in postmenopausal women on combined oestrogen and progesterone preparations
(c) Is usually (in over 50% of cases) a squamous carcinoma
(d) Is best treated by simple hysterectomy with conservation of the ovaries in early cases
(e) May be diagnosed by cervical cytology in 25–30% of cases

83 Stage I carcinoma of the endometrium:

(a) Is best managed by vaginal hysterectomy
(b) Is confined to the uterus
(c) Will have spread to the lymph nodes in approximately 10% of patients
(d) Is the commonest stage at the time of diagnosis
(e) Should be treated with postoperative radiotherapy

80 (a) **True** Stage I may be further divided into stages IA and IB, but these are both confined to the cervix of the uterus.
  (b) **True** This is stage IA.
  (c) **False** Spread to lymph nodes is more common. The 5-year corrected survival rates are 75% for stage I cancer of the cervix, and 90% for endometrial cancer.
  (d) **False** This would be classified as stage III, as staging takes into account normal preoperative investigations.
  (e) **True** The radiation dose decreases according to the inverse square law, and therefore separate internal and external doses are required to cover local lesion and pelvic nodes.

81 (a) **True** However, this is very rare with modern treatment in the absence of a recurrence, but if tumour has eroded the bladder prior to treatment it is more likely.
  (b) **True** Secretions may accumulate behind a fibrotic and stenosed cervix.
  (c) **True** This is the commonest side-effect. It is treated with steroid suppositories.
  (d) **False**
  (e) **True** This is inevitable, unless the ovaries are surgically transposed.

82 (a) **False** Although the peak incidence is between the ages of 50 and 65 years, 20–25% of cases occur premenopausally.
  (b) **False** Unopposed natural oestrogen (from granulosa cell tumours, polycystic ovary syndrome) or exogenous oestrogen predisposes to cancer of the endometrium, whereas combined therapy does not. Indeed, there is now evidence that it is protective against this disease.
  (c) **False** It is usually adenocarcinoma, or occasionally a mixture of adeno- and squamous carcinoma.
  (d) **False** The ovaries are a common site for metastases, and oestrogen secretion activates any residual cancer cells.
  (e) **True** Although it may be picked up on cervical cytology, a negative smear does not preclude the diagnosis of endometrial carcinoma.

83 (a) **False** This procedure should only be used if the patient is a very poor operative risk, and it is usually followed by radiotherapy.
  (b) **False** It is confined to the *body* of the uterus. If the cervix is involved, it is classed as stage II. This is in contrast to cancer of the cervix, which is stage I provided that it is confined to the uterus as a whole.
  (c) **True** This is why lymph-node biopsy is important.
  (d) **True** About 80% of cases are stage I.
  (e) **False** Only cases with poor prognostic features (e.g. deep myometrial invasion or poor differentiation) should be treated thus.

84 Radiotherapy for cancer of the cervix:

(a) May be curative

(b) Has approximately the same success rate as Wertheim's hysterectomy for stage I lesions of the ectocervix

(c) Should not be used after a Wertheim's hysterectomy

(d) May consist of two intracavity caesium applications followed by external irradiation to the pelvic side-walls

(e) Can be repeated if the tumour recurs after the initial standard dose (5000–8000 cGy)

85 Curative radiotherapy for gynaecological malignancy:

(a) Is dependent mainly on beta-rays

(b) May consist of intracavity radium or caesium and external radiation from supervoltage X-ray machines or cobalt

(c) May involve intracavity cobalt

(d) May be repeated after 2 years for a local recurrence

(e) Is potentiated by hypoxia

84 (a) **True** For example, 80–90% of stage I ectocervical cancers can be cured by this treatment.
   (b) **True** This has been confirmed by several large studies.
   (c) **False** If cancerous lymph nodes are removed, irradiation to the pelvic side-walls is often used.
   (d) **True** This is the widely used Manchester technique for cancer of the cervix.
   (e) **False** The maximum dose of radiation that tissues will tolerate is 8000 cGy, which cannot be repeated.

85 (a) **False** It is dependent on gamma-rays; beta-rays (electrons or positrons) and alpha-particles are screened out.
   (b) **True** This would be the standard radiotherapy regime for carcinoma of the cervix.
   (c) **True** Cobalt is usually used for external irradiation, but a machine known as the cathetron can be used to administer intracavity cobalt irradiation.
   (d) **False** This has a high risk of causing extensive necrosis and fistula formation.
   (e) **False** The reverse is true.

MALIGNANT DISEASE OF THE OVARY

86 The following substances may be secreted by ovarian tumours:

(a) Thyroid-stimulating hormone (TSH)
(b) Serotonin
(c) Calmodulin
(d) Chorionic gonadotrophin
(e) Vaso-active intestinal peptide

87 The following ovarian tumours are always malignant:

(a) Myxoma peritonei
(b) Endodermal sinus tumour
(c) Solid teratoma
(d) Granulosa cell tumours
(e) Brenner tumours

88 Mucin-secreting neoplasms of the ovary:

(a) Are usually malignant
(b) Are usually unilocular
(c) Can usually be differentiated from single follicular cysts by ultrasound
(d) Are more often bilateral than other ovarian tumours
(e) Should always be removed

89 Carcinoma of the ovary:

(a) Has a good prognosis if the capsule of the ovary has not been penetrated
(b) Is aggravated by oestrogens
(c) Is classified as stage II if it has spread to the pelvic peritoneum
(d) Typically spreads across the peritoneal cavity
(e) Frequently causes intestinal obstruction

86 (a) **False** Thyroxine, not TSH, is secreted by the *Struma ovarii* of a dermoid cyst.

(b) **True** Carcinoid syndrome may result.

(c) **False** This is an intracellular substance. However, hypercalcaemia may occur due to parathormone or prostaglandin secretion.

(d) **True** This is an important 'tumour marker' in choriocarcinoma and endodermal sinus tumour.

(e) **False** Although these peptides may affect the production of various ovarian steroids *in vivo*, they have not been shown to be produced by tumours.

87 (a) **False** Although spread of benign mucinous cells through the peritoneal cavity is a very serious disorder leading to cachexia, it cannot be regarded as a malignant tumour.

(b) **True** Potentially this is the most malignant tumour in the human body, but the prognosis has been transformed by chemotherapy.

(c) **False** If mature tissues predominate, it is benign.

(d) **False** Only about 30% of these tumours are malignant. However, malignant potential cannot be reliably predicted from histological appearance.

(e) **False** These tumours are nearly always benign.

88 (a) **False** Only 5–10% are malignant.

(b) **False**

(c) **True** The loculi show up on ultrasound.

(d) **False** Only 5% are bilateral, whilst 50% of serous cystadenocarcinomas are bilateral.

(e) **True** Unlike simple functional cysts, all neoplasms of the ovary should be removed in order to exclude malignancy and prevent complications such as torsion or rupture.

89 (a) **True** Unfortunately, ovarian cancer is seldom detected at this early stage. Occasionally, however, such stage IA tumours are discovered by chance at laparotomy for other reasons.

(b) **False** It is seldom if ever hormone responsive.

(c) **True** Stage II implies spread within the pelvis.

(d) **True** This is the commonest mode of spread.

(e) **True** This is a frequent terminal complication.

90 Malignant ovarian disease:

(a) Is the commonest cause of death from cancer of the reproductive tract in the UK
(b) Is usually (FIGO) stage IV when it is discovered
(c) Is staged at operation, unlike cancer of the cervix, which is staged preoperatively
(d) Often presents with amenorrhoea in premenopausal patients
(e) Is more common in women who have never been pregnant

91 In the management of cancer of the ovary:

(a) Chemotherapy is more effective than with other epithelial tumours
(b) Progesterone administration may cause a temporary remission
(c) Extensive surgery has no place in (FIGO) stage III carcinoma
(d) Dysgerminomas are effectively treated by radiotherapy
(e) Radiotherapy has a very limited place

92 Midline incisions are inferior to lower transverse incisions for gynaecological operations in the following respects:

(a) Exposure is less adequate
(b) Incisional hernia is more common
(c) Dehiscence of the scar is more likely
(d) Wound haematoma is more common
(e) The cosmetic result is worse.

90 (a) **True** However, it is not the commonest malignancy of the
reproductive organs.
  (b) **False** It is usually stage III. However, this denotes abdominal spread
beyond the pelvic cavity and the prognosis is usually poor.
  (c) **True** Laparotomy is the only method of determining the absolute
extent of spread.
  (d) **False** Only the rare androgen-secreting tumours cause amenorrhoea
at an early stage.
  (e) **True** There is an association with low or nil parity.

91 (a) **True**
  (b) **False** Endometrial carcinoma may have hormone receptors and
respond temporarily to progesterone treatment.
  (c) **False** Removal of the bulk of the tumour mass increases the
response rate of chemotherapy.
  (d) **True** They are sensitive to radiotherapy in the same way as
seminomas, which they resemble histologically.
  (e) **True** It is useful for the rare dysgerminoma, and rarely for stage II
disease.

92 (a) **False** It is better and the incision may easily be extended.
  (b) **True** The rectus sheath should be repaired with a non-absorbable
material to lower the incidence of this complication after
midline incisions.
  (c) **True** Dehiscence of low transverse incisions is almost unknown.
  (d) **False** The large exposed areas behind the rectus sheath and on the
surface of the rectus abdominus muscles predispose to
haematoma formation. The wound is often drained for this
reason.
  (e) **True** The incision cuts across Lange's lines, and therefore leaves a
wider scar.

MALIGNANT DISEASE OF THE OVARY

CONDITIONS AFFECTING THE VULVA AND VAGINA

93 The following vulval conditions cause pruritus vulvae:

(a) Hypertrophic dystrophy
(b) Lymphogranuloma venereum
(c) Condylomata acuminata
(d) Syphilitic chancre
(e) Threadworms

94 Bartholin's cysts:

(a) Should always be excised to prevent recurrence.
(b) Are situated on the inner side of the posterior end of the labium majus
(c) May become infected by gonorrhoea
(d) Are usually bilateral
(e) May be easily confused with hidradenoma

95 Carcinoma of the vulva:

(a) Does not ulcerate until it is advanced
(b) Is usually histologically anaplastic
(c) Spreads initially to iliac nodes via vaginal lymphatics
(d) Seldom involves lymph nodes at the time of presentation
(e) Is equally amenable to treatment by surgery and radiotherapy

93 (a) **True** The diagnosis is only made after biopsy, which will establish the degree of cellular atypia, and hence the risk of malignancy developing.
(b) **False** The ulcers are characteristically painless.
(c) **True** Vulval warts may be intensely itchy.
(d) **False** Chancre is classically painless and non-irritant.
(e) **True** In children the migration of anal threadworms may cause vulval irritation.

94 (a) **False** Marsupialization is the primary treatment of choice, as it is a smaller operation and preserves the function of the gland.
(b) **True** A cyst in the anterior part of the labium majus may be a cyst of the canal of Nuck.
(c) **True** The vulval and vaginal skin is resistant to gonococcal infection, but Bartholin's glands, Skene's glands and the cervix may be infected.
(d) **False** It is unusual to see simultaneous bilateral cysts, but sometimes a contralateral cyst develops at a later date.
(e) **False** Hidradenoma is a small (< 2 cm), solid, benign tumour of sweat glands.

95 (a) **False** Ulceration is usually an early sign.
(b) **False** It is usually well differentiated.
(c) **False** Spread is to the inguinal nodes.
(d) **False** These lymph nodes are involved in 50% of cases at presentation.
(e) **False** The surrounding tissues will not tolerate effective doses of radiotherapy.

IMAGING IN GYNAECOLOGY

96 The following are readily diagnosed on pelvic ultrasound:

(a) Uterine fibroids
(b) Adenomyosis
(c) Ovarian cancer
(d) Polycystic ovarian syndrome
(e) Hydrosalpinx

97 Early pregnancy ultrasound:

(a) The gestational sac can be seen 3 weeks after conception on transvaginal ultrasound
(b) The yolk sac should be visible at 6 weeks after the last menstrual period (LMP)
(c) If the serum βHCG is > 500 IU, then a gestational sac should be visible
(d) If the sac diameter is > 15 mm, an embryo should be visible
(e) Fetal heart motion may not be seen until the crown–rump length (CRL) is 5 mm

96 (a) **True** The site (submucous, subserous, mural) and size are readily delineated.
   (b) **False** Although adenomyosis may be identified, it is not readily diagnosed.
   (c) **False** Malignancy may only be suspected, and diagnosis requires histology.
   (d) **False** Polycystic ovaries, not the syndrome, are diagnosed on ultrasound.
   (e) **True** Hydrosalpinges, secondary to chronic pelvic infection, are easily identified.

97 (a) **True** This is equivalent to 5 weeks after the LMP.
   (b) **True** The presence of a yolk sac is a good prognostic sign for the pregnancy.
   (c) **False** A gestational sac may not be seen until the βHCG is > 1000 IU.
   (d) **False** The average sac diameter is 20 mm when the embryo is visible.
   (e) **False** The CRL is usually 7–8 mm when fetal heart activity is seen.

INFECTIONS IN GYNAECOLOGY

98 The vulva:

(a) May be the site of primary *Trichomonas* infection
(b) Is the site of 5% of all malignant growths of the female reproductive tract
(c) Becomes atrophic after the menopause
(d) May be the site of lichen sclerosis et atrophicus
(e) May be involved in primary, secondary and tertiary syphilis

99 *Candida* infection has a recognized association with:

(a) Oral contraception
(b) Chronic renal disease
(c) Antibiotic treatment
(d) The menopause
(e) Cervical dysplasia

100 Bacterial vaginosis:

(a) Is the commonest cause of vaginal discharge
(b) Is commoner in women with an IUCD *in situ*
(c) Is associated with an increase in the vaginal pH and the number of anaerobes
(d) Is diagnosed by the presence of 'clue cells' on microscopy
(e) Causative organisms include *Gardnerella*, *Bacteroides* and *Lactobacillus*

101 *Trichomonas*:

(a) Can be asymptomatic for several months after it has been acquired
(b) Is characterized by a purulent offensive discharge and a 'tomato' cervix
(c) Light-background microscopy readily identifies the multiflagellate organism
(d) Usually coexists with bacterial vaginosis
(e) Management is usually with metronidazole and contact tracing

98 (a) **False** It is a *vaginal* infection.
   (b) **True** It most commonly occurs in the elderly.
   (c) **True** The degree to which atrophy occurs is very variable, and hormone replacement therapy (HRT) prevents this.
   (d) **True** Hyperkeratosis is the feature that distinguishes it from primary atrophy, and pruritis is often intense.
   (e) **True** Gumma formation may occur in tertiary syphilis, condylomata lata in secondary disease and chancre in primary syphilis.

99 (a) **True** The oral contraceptive pill probably induces subtle changes in the vaginal flora or pH which increase susceptibility to *Candida* infection.
   (b) **False**
   (c) **True** This commonly precedes *Candida* infection, because it alters the vaginal flora.
   (d) **False** Loss of glycogen from vaginal epithelium occurs at the menopause, and vaginal *Candida* infection becomes less likely.
   (e) **False** This is in contrast to the typical sexually transmitted infections, such as *Trichomonas* and papilloma virus.

100 (a) **True** In women of reproductive age.
    (b) **True** It is commoner in women with IUCDs.
    (c) **True** It is caused by overgrowth of vaginal commensals.
    (d) **True** And addition of alkali to discharge produces a characteristic 'fishy' odour.
    (e) **False** *Lactobacillus* is not a causative organism.

101 (a) **True** Symptoms may occur several months after sexual intercourse.
    (b) **False** Punctate haemorrhages of the cervix give a 'strawberry' appearance.
    (c) **False** Dark-background microscopy is required for this test.
    (d) **True**
    (e) **True**

102 *Chlamydia trachomatis*:

- (a) Is usually asymptomatic
- (b) Can also infect the throat and conjunctiva
- (c) Differs from other bacteria in that it is an intracellular pathogen
- (d) Is diagnosed on high vaginal swabs
- (e) May be treated with doxycycline, erythromycin or azithromycin

103 Gonorrhoea:

- (a) Women are more likely to be symptomatic than men
- (b) *Neisseria gonorrhoea* is a Gram-negative diplococcus
- (c) Gonorrhoea is increasingly resistant to penicillins and quinolones
- (d) Vaginal swabs are adequate for diagnosis
- (e) In over 50% of cases women are also infected with chlamydia

104 Genital warts:

- (a) The majority of genital warts are caused by human papilloma virus (HPV) types 6 and 11
- (b) The same HPV types (6 and 11) have been linked to the development of cervical cancer
- (c) Genital warts may be treated with cryotherapy or podophyllin
- (d) Infections may last for many years with relapses at any time
- (e) *Molluscum contagiosum* is a pox virus that can occur spontaneously in childhood

105 HIV infection:

- (a) The incidence of HIV worldwide is now levelling off
- (b) Infected individuals show symptoms within 10 years
- (c) The principal mode of spread is vaginal intercourse
- (d) Anti-retroviral therapy reduces hospitalization but not life expectancy
- (e) Genital warts, cervical and vulval intra-epithelial neoplasia are common presentations

102 (a) **True** In 50% of men and 80% of women.
    (b) **False** It may cause conjunctivitus and colonize, but not infect, the throat.
    (c) **True** It enters cells by binding to specific cell-surface receptors.
    (d) **False** Endocervical swabs are required, as live columnar cells are harvested.
    (e) **True** Treatment of sexual partners is mandatory.

103 (a) **False** 90% of men and 50% of women are symptomatic.
    (b) **True**
    (c) **True** Treatment is dictated by local sensitivity patterns.
    (d) **False** Vaginal, urethral and rectal swabs should be taken for culture.
    (e) **True** Chlamydia treatment is routinely prescribed for these women and their partners.

104 (a) **True** These are sexually transmitted.
    (b) **False** HPV types 16 and 18 are linked to cervical cancer.
    (c) **True** Podophyllin requires twice weekly application for 6 weeks.
    (d) **True** Recent partners, although at risk, may not have been the source of infection.
    (e) **True** It is common in childhood, infectious, and resolves spontaneously.

105 (a) **False** The incidence is increasing rapidly worldwide.
    (b) **False** Infected individuals may remain well for 15–20 years.
    (c) **True** In developed countries, homosexual sex and intravenous drug use are important routes.
    (d) **False** Anti-retroviral therapy reduces hospitalization and increases life expectancy.
    (e) **True**

INCONTINENCE

106 Incontinence of urine:

(a) Is commonly caused by prolapse
(b) May be caused by diabetes mellitus
(c) May be due to overflow incontinence in multiple sclerosis
(d) May be congenital
(e) Is best treated surgically if detrusor instability is the cause

107 Stress incontinence of urine:

(a) Is more common in multiparous patients
(b) Can be controlled by para-urethral pressure during vaginal examination
(c) Can be differentiated from urge incontinence by means of a cystometrogram
(d) Should be investigated by cystoscopy prior to surgery
(e) May be a transient problem after delivery

108 Treatment of genuine stress incontinence:

(a) 20% of women will show satisfactory improvement of symptoms with pelvic floor exercises
(b) The purpose of surgery is to restore the anatomical position of the proximal urethra
(c) Periurethral injections are of particular value when surgery has failed
(d) A urodynamics investigation is not mandatory before surgery is undertaken
(e) Surgery is advisable, as it cannot worsen the symptoms

106 (a) **False** It is associated with but not caused by prolapse.
   (b) **True** Diabetic neuropathy may lead to *overflow* incontinence, as with other lower motor neurone lesions.
   (c) **False** This causes high-pressure, urge incontinence as with other upper motor neurone lesions.
   (d) **True** Occasionally a ureter may drain directly into the vagina.
   (e) **False** Surgery is reserved for genuine stress incontinence.

107 (a) **True** Childbirth is the most important aetiological factor.
   (b) **True** This is called Bonney's test.
   (c) **True** Surgical operations for stress incontinence should not be performed unless urodynamic tests have confirmed the diagnosis.
   (d) **False** Cystoscopy has little place in the evaluation of incontinence.
   (e) **True** Surgery should only be considered if incontinence persists for 3 months after delivery.

108 (a) **False** Around 40–60% of women will only require this therapy.
   (b) **True** Surgery may also increase urethral resistance.
   (c) **True** Previous surgery does not make this technique difficult, unlike repeat surgery.
   (d) **False** Urodynamics will determine the need for surgery and the type of operation.
   (e) **False** Any detrusor instability may be worsened by surgery.

PROLAPSE

109 Uterovaginal prolapse:

(a) Is a very painful condition
(b) Is commonly worse in the erect position
(c) The cervix is often elongated
(d) Is common in Afro-Caribbean women
(e) May cause intestinal obstruction if there is a large rectocele

110 An enterocele:

(a) Is a prolapse of the rectum
(b) May occur following a colposuspension
(c) Should initially be treated with a shelf pessary
(d) May resolve spontaneously
(e) Is a common cause of stress incontinence

111 Retroversion of the uterus:

(a) Occurs in 15% of normal women
(b) Is a common cause of infertility
(c) May be corrected by a Fothergill operation
(d) Is caused by heavy lifting
(e) Should always be corrected with a Hodge pessary in early pregnancy

112 Cystocele:

(a) Is a prolapse of the bladder and anterior vaginal wall
(b) Is common after the menopause
(c) Is the cause of stress incontinence of urine
(d) May lead to urinary infection
(e) Is very uncommon in nulliparous women

109 (a) **False** There is rarely pain, even with gross degrees of prolapse.
   (b) **True** Lying down almost always relieves prolapse.
   (c) **True** Elongation of the supravaginal cervix occurs with major degrees of uterine prolapse.
   (d) **False** It is strikingly uncommon in this group.
   (e) **False** Difficulty in defaecation may occur, but not obstruction.

110 (a) **False** It is a hernia of the pouch of Douglas, and therefore at a higher level than the rectum.
   (b) **True** Colposuspension alters the vaginal angle, potentially leading to hernia of the pouch of Douglas.
   (c) **False** This treatment should only be used in the frail and elderly, or in recurrent cases.
   (d) **False** No conservative measures improve enterocele.
   (e) **False** Unless there is associated anterior vaginal prolapse, stress incontinence will not occur.

111 (a) **True** Provided that the retroversion is mobile, it is of little clinical significance.
   (b) **False** It is only associated with infertility if there is an underlying cause such as endometriosis or chronic pelvic infection.
   (c) **False** The operation to correct retroversion is a ventrosuspension.
   (d) **False** It is either congenital, acquired following childbirth, or secondary to pelvic adhesions.
   (e) **False** A retroverted uterus only rarely becomes incarcerated in pregnancy, and correction with a Hodge pessary is hardly ever indicated.

112 (a) **True** It may or may not be accompanied by uterine or other vaginal prolapse.
   (b) **True** Oestrogen deficiency results in atrophy of the supporting fascia.
   (c) **False** Stress incontinence is often associated with cystocele, but is not caused by it.
   (d) **True** Stasis of urine from any cause may lead to infection.
   (e) **True** It is almost always a consequence of childbirth.

113 Anterior colporrhaphy:

(a) May cause temporary retention of urine
(b) Is commonly used in the treatment of stress incontinence
(c) Is frequently combined with vaginal hysterectomy
(d) Should be avoided in patients with urge incontinence
(e) Should not be performed until childbearing is complete

113 (a) **True** Routine postoperative catheterization, preferably with a suprapubic catheter, is often used for this purpose.

    (b) **False** Colposuspension and sling procedures have a higher success rate, and are more frequently used today.

    (c) **True**

    (d) **True** It may make matters worse.

    (e) **False** However, most surgeons would recommend delivery by Caesarean section after successful anterior colporrhaphy.

MENOPAUSE

MENOPAUSE

114 After the menopause:

(a) There is a reduction in vaginal acidity
(b) Gonadotrophin secretion decreases
(c) Any vaginal bleeding should be investigated by an endometrial biopsy/D & C
(d) Treatment with oestrogen is often beneficial
(e) The rate of bone loss is greatest during the first two years

115 Premature ovarian failure:

(a) Is ovarian failure that occurs before 50 years of age
(b) The ovary appears postmenopausal histologically
(c) Is also known as 'resistant ovary syndrome'
(d) Climacteric symptoms are infrequent
(e) Is commonly associated with autoimmune diseases

116 Hormone replacement therapy:

(a) Does not require a physical examination before prescription
(b) Cannot be delivered by the transdermal route
(c) Requires cyclical progestagens even in women without a uterus
(d) Irregular vaginal bleeding is a common symptom which may be ignored
(e) May be prescribed to women with ovarian cancer

114 (a) **True** This may give rise to vaginitis.
   (b) **False** There is an increase in FSH and LH production due to the loss of the oestrogen 'negative feedback'.
   (c) **True** It is essential to exclude carcinoma of the endometrium.
   (d) **True** Atrophic vaginitis is a common cause of dryness and discomfort which can be relieved with oestrogen administered either locally or systemically.
   (e) **True**

115 (a) **False** The definition is under 45 years of age.
   (b) **True**
   (c) **False** In this condition the ovary appears normal histologically.
   (d) **False** These symptoms are often severe.
   (e) **True** In over 50% of cases.

116 (a) **False** Oestrogen-sensitive tumours in the breast or pelvis must be excluded before treatment.
   (b) **False** HRT may be given orally, transdermally or by subcutaneous implants.
   (c) **False** Progestagens are required to prevent endometrial hyperplasia.
   (d) **False** Although it is relatively common, this symptom must be taken seriously.
   (e) **True** This is not an oestrogen-sensitive tumour.

PSYCHOLOGICAL ASPECTS OF GYNAECOLOGY

117 The phases of the female sexual response cycle:

    (a) Include desire
    (b) Include arousal
    (c) Include plateau
    (d) There are five phases
    (e) Are shorter than in the male sexual response cycle

118 Chronic pelvic pain:

    (a) Is a common symptom presenting in gynaecology outpatients
    (a) Laparoscopy detects pathology in 50% of cases
    (a) Identification of pelvic pathology excludes a psychogenic cause
    (a) Avoidance/conflict related to sex and intimacy is a common co-symptom
    (a) Cases should be sent for psychotherapy without investigation

117 (a) **True** There are four phases, namely desire, arousal, orgasm, resolution.
    (b) **True** It is the second phase.
    (c) **False**
    (d) **False**
    (e) **False** The female cycle is longer, and it also lengthens with age.

118 (a) **True**
    (b) **False** Pathology is seen in less than 30% of cases.
    (c) **False** Pelvic pathology may often coexist without being the cause of the pain.
    (d) **True** This would indicate a psychogenic cause.
    (e) **False** A proportion of cases will be due to conditions such as endometriosis or chronic pelvic infection.

PSYCHOLOGICAL ASPECTS OF GYNAECOLOGY

CHAPTER TWO

Obstetric MCQs

OBSTETRIC HISTORY AND EXAMINATION

1 The following associations are appropriate:

(a) Lie: cephalic
(b) Presentation: flexed
(c) Station: at the level of the spines
(d) Engagement: two-fifths palpable
(e) Presenting part: shoulder

2 With regard to pregnancy dating:

(a) The last menstrual period (LMP) is used in preference to ultrasound
(b) The LMP is reliable even if cycles are irregular
(c) The LMP can be used if pregnancy was due to a contraceptive pill failure
(d) Breastfeeding makes LMP dating inaccurate
(e) The EDD is calculated as LMP + 12 months − 3 months + 7 days

3 Gravidity and parity:

(a) Gravidity records the total number of pregnancies excluding the current one
(b) Parity refers to the number of livebirths and stillbirths after 24 weeks
(c) A pregnant woman with a previous 10-week termination would be G2 P0^{+1}
(d) A pregnant woman could be G2 P3
(e) Are not really clinically relevant

1 (a) **False** Cephalic describes presentation.
   (b) **False** Flexion describes the attitude. Presentation would be cephalic/breech.
   (c) **True** Indicates that the presenting part has reached the ischial spines.
   (d) **True** For descriptive purposes the fetal head is divided into fifths.
   (e) **True** The shoulder can present with a transverse lie.

2 (a) **True** Unless there is a significant discrepancy between the two dates.
   (b) **False** Cycles need to be regular and of normal length
   (c) **False** The contraceptive pill induces withdrawal bleeds and not a menstrual bleed.
   (d) **True** The time of ovulation is unpredictable, even if the woman is menstruating while breastfeeding.
   (e) **True** This is termed Nägele's rule.

3 (a) **False** Gravidity includes the current pregnancy.
   (b) **False** Parity includes livebirths irrespective of gestation and stillbirths after 24 weeks.
   (c) **True** See above definition of parity (b).
   (d) **True** If she had triplets in her last pregnancy.
   (e) **False** Many obstetric risk factors are related to parity and gravidity.

MATERNAL AND PERINATAL MORTALITY

4   Maternal mortality:

(a) Now stands at a rate of less than 0.1 per 1000 total births
(b) Does not include deaths from therapeutic abortion
(c) Must be reported to the Coroner
(d) Is subjected to a Confidential Enquiry
(e) Is most often caused by sepsis

5   Perinatal mortality:

(a) Includes all stillbirths
(b) Includes all neonatal deaths in the first month of life
(c) Is increased in social classes 4 and 5
(d) Is higher for mothers aged under 20 years than for those over 35 years
(e) The perinatal mortality rate is around 1 per 1000 total births

6   CESDI:

(a) Stands for Confidential Enquiry into Sudden Deaths in Infancy
(b) Includes only deaths after 24 weeks' gestation
(c) Late neonatal deaths occur after the first month of life
(d) Is principally caused by congenital abnormality
(e) Was set up to investigate suboptimal medical care

4 (a) **True** The rate has fallen to this level from a rate of 4 per 1000 in 1928.

   (b) **False** Deaths from abortion (either spontaneous or therapeutic) are included.

   (c) **False** The same regulations relate to reporting to the Coroner as with any type of death.

   (d) **True** This is a national audit which has done much to focus attention on areas where standards of care can be improved.

   (e) **False** Thromboembolic disease is the commonest cause, followed by hypertensive disease.

5 (a) **True** Stillbirths at any gestation are included.

   (b) **False** Only early neonatal deaths (in the first week of life) are included.

   (c) **True**

   (d) **False** However, both groups have an increased risk of perinatal mortality.

   (e) **False** The rate is approximately 8.7 per 1000 total births in the UK.

6 (a) **False** It stands for Confidential Enquiry into Stillbirths and Deaths in Infancy.

   (b) **False** It includes deaths after 20 weeks' gestation.

   (c) **False** Late neonatal deaths occur from 7 to 27 completed days after birth.

   (d) **False** The principal cause is prematurity, followed by congenital abnormality.

   (e) **True** The report classifies cases according to the type of care that they received.

EARLY PREGNANCY – CONCEPTION, IMPLANTATION AND EMBRYOLOGY

7   During the development of ovarian follicles:

   (a) The first polar body is extruded before ovulation
   (b) Meiosis is resumed 1 week before ovulation
   (c) The ovum is extruded at the peak of the LH surge
   (d) Progesterone secretion starts to increase before ovulation
   (e) Granulosa cells in the corpus luteum are responsible for steroidogenesis

8   The luteal phase of the menstrual cycle is associated with:

   (a) High progesterone levels
   (b) High LH levels
   (c) Low basal body temperature
   (d) Implantation
   (e) Rising FSH levels

9   Meiosis and mitosis:

   (a) Most human cells contain 44 autosomes
   (b) Mature sperm contain 23 chromosomes
   (c) Mitosis is a two-stage process
   (d) Meiosis produces haploid eggs or sperm
   (e) The ovum determines the sex of the child

7 (a) **True** The primary oocyte divides by meiosis while it is still in the ovary.
  (b) **False** It is resumed 36–48 hours after the peak and 36 hours after the start of the LH surge.
  (c) **False** Ovulation occurs 12 hours after the peak and 36 hours after the start of the LH surge.
  (d) **True** It does not peak until 7 days after ovulation, but it begins to rise well before it.
  (e) **True** They become granulosa lutein cells, and provide steroids.

8 (a) **True** Progesterone levels reach a peak at mid-luteal phase.
  (b) **False** The LH peak occurs prior to ovulation.
  (c) **False** The basal temperature rises after ovulation.
  (d) **True** The blastocyst starts to implant 7 days after ovulation.
  (e) **False** The FSH level rises in the follicular phase.

9 (a) **True** Cells contain 46 chromosomes (44 autosomes and 2 sex chromosomes).
  (b) **True** This is a haploid cell.
  (c) **False** Meiosis is a two-stage process.
  (d) **True**
  (e) **False** The sperm may contain either an X-chromosome or a Y-chromosome, thereby determining the sex.

EARLY PREGNANCY – CONCEPTION, IMPLANTATION AND EMBRYOLOGY

PHYSIOLOGICAL CHANGES IN PREGNANCY

10 Maternal blood flow to the placenta:

(a) Reaches about 1000 mL per minute by the end of pregnancy
(b) Is affected by posture
(c) Is completely obstructed during the peak of strong contractions
(d) Is reduced in pre-eclampsia
(e) Is increased by inspiration of 100% oxygen

11 Maternal cardiovascular and haematological changes:

(a) The red cell mass decreases
(b) The haemoglobin concentration and white cell count decrease
(c) The erythrocyte sedimentation rate increases
(d) The stroke volume increases
(e) The peripheral resistance and mean arterial pressure decrease

12 During normal pregnancy:

(a) Estradiol is the principal circulating oestrogen
(b) The blood pressure falls in the second trimester
(c) Blood flow to the liver and kidneys increases by over 25%
(d) The pressure of the uterus on the diaphragm reduces the tidal volume and causes dyspnoea
(e) The ureters dilate due to obstruction and increased intraluminal pressure

13 Fibroids in pregnancy:

(a) Are a recognized cause of obstructed labour
(b) Should be removed by myomectomy during pregnancy
(c) Should be removed by myomectomy at Caesarean section
(d) Are likely to regress after the pregnancy
(e) May cause acute abdominal pain

10 (a) **True**
   (b) **True** The pressure of the uterus on the inferior vena cava in the supine position obstructs venous return to the heart (supine hypotension).
   (c) **True** Venules in the myometrium are completely occluded by the surrounding muscle fibres.
   (d) **True** This is an important component of the pathophysiology of pre-eclampsia.
   (e) **False** There is some evidence that it may be decreased, but none that it is increased.

11 (a) **False** However, as the plasma volume increases, the haemoglobin concentration falls.
   (b) **False** The white cell count increases in pregnancy.
   (c) **True**
   (d) **True** The stroke volume increases by approximately 10%.
   (e) **True** The arterial pressure falls because of a reduction in peripheral vascular resistance.

12 (a) **False** Estriol is the principal oestrogen.
   (b) **True** The diastolic pressure is reduced in both the first and second trimesters.
   (c) **False** Blood flow to the kidneys increases by 30% but hepatic flow remains unchanged.
   (d) **False** The tidal volume is increased due to the effect of progesterone on the respiratory centre.
   (e) **False** Dilation is due to the smooth muscle relaxant effect of progesterone.

13 (a) **True** Fibroids situated in the pelvis may rarely obstruct labour.
   (b) **False** Abortion/haemorrhage is likely if myomectomy is attempted during pregnancy.
   (c) **False** Again, dangerous haemorrhage may occur.
   (d) **True** Fibroids are oestrogen-dependent tumours.
   (e) **True** Degeneration of fibroids is common in pregnancy, causing severe pain.

14 The uterus and cervix in pregnancy:

(a) Uterine growth is by hypertrophy only
(b) The lower uterine segment forms at 20 weeks
(c) Infrequent painful contractions are termed 'Braxton–Hicks' contractions
(d) Cervical ectropion is seen more frequently
(e) Prostaglandins are produced in the cervix

15 Retroversion of the uterus in pregnancy:

(a) Is a common cause of recurrent abortion
(b) May cause acute retention of urine
(c) Should be corrected by the insertion of a Hodge pessary
(d) Usually corrects itself spontaneously after week 12
(e) Is often associated with stress incontinence

14 (a) **False** Hypertrophy and hyperplasia both contribute towards uterine growth in pregnancy.

(b) **False** The lower segment forms in the late second trimester. It extends from the peritoneum of the uterovesical pouch superiorly to the internal cervical os inferiorly.

(c) **False** These contractions are painless and reflect the maturation of cellular gap junctions.

(d) **True** The cervical columnar epithelium is oestrogen-dependent.

(e) **True** They are produced increasingly towards term.

15 (a) **False** This misconception was abandoned many years ago.

(b) **True** It causes retention between weeks 12 and 16.

(c) **False** This is not generally necessary, as the retroversion corrects itself.

(d) **True** Only very rarely does incarceration occur.

(e) **False** If incarceration occurs, urinary retention with overflow incontinence occurs.

PHYSIOLOGICAL CHANGES IN PREGNANCY

NORMAL FETAL DEVELOPMENT AND GROWTH

16 Fetal size:

(a) The average weight at term is 3 kg
(b) Size is increased in multiparous women
(c) Male infants are usually smaller than female infants
(d) Size is increased in heavier mothers
(e) Smoking 10 cigarettes a day decreases birth-weight by an average of 100 g

17 Fetal development:

(a) Fetal haematopoiesis starts in the bone marrow at 6 weeks
(b) Fetal breathing movements occur before birth
(c) The immune system is undeveloped, relying on passive immune protection
(d) Fetal movements begin from around 18 weeks
(e) Amniotic fluid is required for normal lung development

18 By the time a fetus is mature it is usual for:

(a) Meconium to have been passed
(b) Pulmonary surfactant to have been produced
(c) The ductus arteriosus to have closed
(d) The hepatic glucuronyl transferase system to be adequate
(e) Fetal haemoglobin to be 16–20 g/100 mL

19 In the fetal circulation:

(a) Oxygenated blood travels along the umbilical arteries
(b) The fetal lungs are bypassed by means of the ductus venosus
(c) The foramen ovale connects the two atria
(d) Most of the blood that enters the right atrium flows into the left atrium
(e) The blood in the descending aorta is more desaturated than that in the ascending aorta

16 (a) **False** The average weight is 3.5 kg.
   (b) **True** Fetal weight usually increases with each pregnancy.
   (c) **False** Male infants are approximately 60 g heavier.
   (d) **False** Maternal height, not weight, is associated with fetal growth.
   (e) **False** Smoking 10 cigarettes a day decreases fetal weight at term by 200 g.

17 (a) **False** Haematopoiesis starts in the liver and spleen at 6 weeks.
   (b) **True** Breathing movements occur increasingly frequently towards term.
   (c) **False** Cellular and humoral immune activity is detectable from 18 weeks.
   (d) **False** Movements begin much earlier, but may not be felt until 18 weeks.
   (e) **True** The absence of amniotic fluid predisposes to pulmonary hypoplasia.

18 (a) **False** If meconium is passed before birth, it is usually a sign of fetal distress.
   (b) **True** This is normally present from weeks 32 to 34 of gestation.
   (c) **False** It usually closes some time after birth.
   (d) **True** The inadequacy of this enzyme system is the cause of physiological jaundice.
   (e) **True** Fetal polycythaemia aids maternal to fetal oxygen transfer.

19 (a) **False** Deoxygenated blood is returned to the placenta via the umbilical arteries.
   (b) **False** It is the ductus arteriosus.
   (c) **True** Blood passes from the right to the left atrium.
   (d) **True** Blood from the inferior vena cava passes through the foramen ovale.
   (e) **True** Mixing with blood from the ductus arteriosus causes the lower oxygen saturation.

NORMAL FETAL DEVELOPMENT AND GROWTH

20 **The fetus:**

(a) Is most vulnerable to teratogenic agents between 10 and 12 weeks
(b) Usually weighs over 1 kg at 28 weeks
(c) Develops recognizable external genitalia at 14 weeks
(d) Can survive hypoxia for longer than an adult
(e) Will develop anaemia if the mother is iron-deficient

20 (a) **False** The most critical period is in the early first trimester – during organogenesis.

(b) **True** The average fetal weight at 28 weeks is 1100 g.

(c) **True** Modern ultrasound equipment will often permit diagnosis of the sex of the fetus at 14 weeks.

(d) **True**

(e) **False** The fetal serum iron concentration will be maintained at the expense of that of the mother.

NORMAL FETAL DEVELOPMENT AND GROWTH

ULTRASOUND IMAGING AND ASSESSMENT OF FETAL WELL-BEING

21 By means of real-time ultrasound examination:

- (a) Pregnancy can usually be detected 5 weeks after the last menstrual period
- (b) The fetal heart cannot be seen until 10 weeks after the last period
- (c) Placenta praevia can be reliably demonstrated at week 16 of pregnancy
- (d) The biparietal diameter can be measured reliably after week 12 of pregnancy
- (e) A reliable estimate of gestational age can be made in the third trimester

22 The following ultrasonic measurements may be used to confirm or establish gestation:

- (a) Crown–rump length
- (b) Biparietal diameter
- (c) Nuchal translucency
- (d) Gestational sac volume
- (e) Yolk sac volume

23 Doppler ultrasound:

- (a) Abnormal uterine Doppler flow indicates fetal hypoxaemia
- (b) Abnormal umbilical artery flow indicates poor placental perfusion
- (c) Fetal anaemia is associated with redistribution of blood flow
- (d) Fetal hypoxaemia is associated with a hyperdynamic circulation
- (e) Abnormal ductus venosus blood flow occurs before arterial changes

24 Normal cardiotocograms (CTGs):

- (a) The baseline at term is usually 120–160 beats/minute
- (b) The short-term variability is 10–25 beats/minute
- (c) An acceleration is a baseline increase of 15 beats/minute for 15 seconds
- (d) A reactive trace would have one acceleration in 20 minutes
- (e) The tocograph trace indicates the strength of contractions

21 (a) **True** Transvaginal ultrasound detects the gestation sac by 5 weeks.
   (b) **False** It can normally be demonstrated at 6–7 weeks.
   (c) **False** The lower segment has not formed; therefore praevia cannot be diagnosed.
   (d) **True** However, the crown–rump length is most accurate between 7 and 12 weeks for dating.
   (e) **False** This is due to the wide range of fetal size for given gestational age at this stage.

22 (a) **True** This is most accurate between 7 and 12 weeks.
   (b) **True** This is the most appropriate measurement between 15 and 20 weeks.
   (c) **False** Increased nuchal translucency is a predictor of possible Down's syndrome.
   (d) **True** This is useful in very early pregnancy.
   (e) **False** The yolk sac is too small and does not correlate well with gestational age.

23 (a) **False** This indicates a higher risk for pre-eclampsia of uteroplacental insufficiency.
   (b) **True**
   (c) **False** Fetal anaemia is associated with a hyperdynamic circulation.
   (d) **False** Fetal hypoxaemia is associated with redistribution of blood flow.
   (e) **False** Abnormal ductus venosus flow is a pre-terminal event.

24 (a) **False** The normal baseline is 110–150 beats/minute.
   (b) **True** This is also known as baseline variability.
   (c) **True**
   (d) **False** To be classified as 'reactive', a trace requires two accelerations in 20 minutes.
   (e) **False** Tocography shows the frequency but not the strength of contractions.

25 Abnormal CTGs:

(a) Short-term variability of < 10 beats/minute for 30 minutes is abnormal
(b) Tachycardia may occur in normal fetuses because of maternal pyrexia
(c) Prolonged bradycardias are suggestive of fetal hypoxaemia
(d) Late decelerations may occur before contractions begin
(e) All CTGs need to be stored for 25 years

26 Fetal tachycardia:

(a) May be the result of previous maternal thyrotoxicosis
(b) Usually has a good prognosis if baseline variability is retained
(c) Is more common after prolonged rupture of the membranes
(d) Seldom exceeds 200 beats/minute
(e) May occur in severe rhesus disease

27 Biophysical profile:

(a) Is a reflection of fetal well-being assessed by Doppler
(b) Is scored out of 12
(c) Amniotic fluid volume is one of the variables included
(d) The presence of breathing movements is a poor sign
(e) Has a lower false-negative rate for fetal hypoxaemia than CTGs

25 (a) **False** This is normal during the sleep phase, usually followed by a reactive CTG.

   (b) **True** Other reasons include fetal hypoxaemia and anaemia.

   (c) **True** Rarely, congenital heart block may cause bradycardias in normoxaemic fetuses.

   (d) **False** Late decelerations occur just after a uterine contraction.

   (e) **True** They are part of the patient record and this is a medico-legal requirement.

26 (a) **True** Long-acting thyroid-stimulating antibodies may still be present.

   (b) **True** Careful monitoring is warranted because tachycardia may occur in hypoxaemia.

   (c) **True** This is due to the resulting amnionitis and pyrexia.

   (d) **True** Only a fetal arrhythmia will exceed this rate.

   (e) **True** A fast flat trace occurs in acute blood loss or chronic anaemia of rhesus disease.

27 (a) **False** The biophysical profile is assessed by ultrasound and CTG/Doppler.

   (b) **False** It is normally scored out of 10 (five variables scored 0 to 2).

   (c) **True**

   (d) **False** Breathing movements may take 30 minutes to manifest and are physiological.

   (e) **True** However, the test has not been taken up widely as it is more difficult to implement.

ANTENATAL CARE

28 Asymptomatic bacteriuria:

   (a) Occurs in 10% of pregnant women
   (b) Turns to infection in most cases if left untreated
   (c) Occurs in patients with renal tract abnormalities
   (d) Is associated with premature delivery
   (e) Causes an increase in the maternal white cell count

29 Smoking in pregnancy is associated with:

   (a) Low birth weight
   (b) Maternal unemployment
   (c) Increased likelihood of childhood respiratory disease
   (d) Decreased incidence of breastfeeding
   (e) Increased likelihood of pre-eclampsia

30 Antenatal care:

   (a) Has been shown categorically to improve pregnancy outcome
   (b) Is essentially a screening process
   (c) Works independently of antenatal education
   (d) Unbooked pregnancies have the worst outcome
   (e) The key to good care is history-taking

31 Routine booking bloods:

   (a) Maternal anaemia is defined as a haemoglobin (Hb) concentration of < 10 g/dL
   (b) If the mother is rubella non-immune, vaccination should be deferred until after birth
   (c) HIV screening is unjustified as the pregnancy outcome is unlikely to be altered
   (d) Toxoplasmosis and cytomegalovirus are routinely screened for
   (e) Hepatitis B screening is now redundant

28 (a) **False** Occurs in less than 5% of women.
(b) **False** It turns to infection in 30% of cases.
(c) **True** It is more likely to occur in these women.
(d) **True**
(e) **False** This occurs with overt infection.

29 (a) **True** Average birthweight is 200 g less in smokers.
(b) **True** Unemployed women are more likely to be smokers.
(c) **True** Most women continue to smoke after the delivery.
(d) **True** Smokers are less likely to breastfeed.
(e) **False** This may occur less frequently in smokers.

30 (a) **False** However, lack of antenatal care has been shown to worsen pregnancy outcome.
(b) **True** Antenatal care involves screening healthy women for pregnancy complications.
(c) **False** Antenatal education cannot be separated from good antenatal care.
(d) **True** Unbooked women unfortunately require antenatal care the most.
(e) **True** The focus of antenatal care is to identify 'high-risk' cases from the history.

31 (a) **False** Maternal anaemia is defined as an Hb concentration of < 11 g/dL.
(b) **True** The rubella vaccine is a live vaccine which should be deferred until after birth.
(c) **False** Maternal health can be improved and vertical transmission of HIV can be reduced.
(d) **False** Routine testing is avoided because of the low prevalence and high false-positive rates.
(e) **False** Hepatitis B is more seroprevalent than HIV.

32 Anaemia in pregnancy:

(a) Is defined as a haemoglobin concentration of 10.0 g/dL or less
(b) May be caused by haemodilution of pregnancy
(c) May be caused by hookworm infestation
(d) When megaloblastic is usually due to vitamin B_{12} deficiency
(e) Is relatively common in multiple pregnancy

33 In iron deficiency anaemia in pregnancy:

(a) The mean corpuscular haemoglobin content (MCH) and the mean corpuscular haemoglobin concentration (MCHC) are both low
(b) The mean corpuscular volume (MCV) is raised
(c) Blood transfusion is indicated if haemoglobin levels fall to below 9.0 g/dL
(d) There is usually a chronic blood loss causing the anaemia
(e) There is an increased risk of pre-eclampsia

32 (a) **False** It is defined as a haemoglobin level of < 11.0 g/dL.
   (b) **True** The plasma volume may increase by ≥ 30%, resulting in a dilutional anaemia.
   (c) **True** This is the commonest cause of anaemia in some parts of the world.
   (d) **False** Megaloblastic anaemia in pregnancy is usually due to folic acid deficiency.
   (e) **True** This is a result of dilution, and increased iron and folate requirements.

33 (a) **True** In beta-thalassaemia, the MCH is low but the MCHC is normal.
   (b) **False** The MCV is low, with hypochromasia.
   (c) **False** Blood transfusion is used if there is insufficient time for iron therapy to work.
   (d) **False** Inadequate dietary iron is the usual cause.
   (e) **False** There is no relationship between anaemia and pre-eclampsia.

LABOUR

34 The fetal head:

(a) Engages by the mento-vertical diameter in face presentations
(b) When engaged, usually presents with the suboccipito-bregmatic diameter
(c) Contains an anterior fontanelle immediately behind the bregma
(d) Has one occipital and two frontal bones
(e) May be felt abdominally after engagement has taken place

35 Symptoms and signs of the onset of labour include:

(a) Braxton–Hicks contractions
(b) Absent fetal movement
(c) Shortening of the cervix
(d) Dilatation of the cervix
(e) Spinnbarkeit

36 Uterine contractions in labour:

(a) Start at the cornu
(b) Involve uterine muscle retraction
(c) Are painful due to ischaemia
(d) Are efficient at 5 mmHg
(e) Are consciously controllable

37 Electronic fetal monitoring in labour:

(a) Shows the normal heart rate to be 110–150 beats/minute
(b) May involve checking the fetal pH
(c) Is mandatory
(d) Looks for short-term variations
(e) Measures uterine activity and fetal heart rate

34 (a) **False** The mento-vertical diameter is associated with brow presentations.
   (b) **True** This is the diameter which engages when the head is well flexed (9.5 cm).
   (c) **False** The bregma is the point in the middle of the anterior fontanelle.
   (d) **True**
   (e) **True** After engagement, two-fifths or less of the head may be felt abdominally.

35 (a) **False** These may be felt throughout pregnancy as painless, irregular contractions.
   (b) **False** The absence of fetal movements should always be regarded with suspicion.
   (c) **True** This is the earliest change in the latent phase of labour.
   (d) **True** However, in a multigravid woman, the cervical os may be dilated 1–2 cm at term.
   (e) **False** This is a change in the cervical mucus seen at ovulation.

36 (a) **True** Electrical traces show that the contraction wave starts near one or the other cornu.
   (b) **True** When the contraction relaxes, some of the shortening of the fibres is maintained.
   (c) **True** The pain is analogous to the pain of myocardial ischaemia.
   (d) **False** Contractions are not palpable when they are less than 20 mmHg, and efficient contractions reach a pressure of 50 mmHg.
   (e) **False** Only the perception of pain may be altered by emotional state.

37 (a) **True** Note that the baseline may normally be higher in preterm fetuses.
   (b) **True** Fetal scalp blood samples for pH may be taken if there are CTG abnormalities.
   (c) **False** Low-risk normal mothers need intermittent auscultation only.
   (d) **True** Lack of short-term variation may indicate fetal hypoxaemia.
   (e) **True** Both uterine activity and fetal heart rate may be measured.

38 Active management of the third stage:

(a) Involves the Matthews–Duncan method
(b) May involve intravenous syntocinon
(c) Increases the risk that a manual removal will be needed
(d) Increases the likelihood of postpartum haemorrhage
(e) Begins with delivery of the fetal trunk

39 The second stage of labour:

(a) Causes a transient bradycardia with contractions which are of little significance
(b) Is less painful than the first
(c) Ends with placental separation
(d) Starts with pushing
(e) Is shorter in multiparae

40 The third stage of labour:

(a) Starts early in the second stage
(b) Ends with placental separation
(c) Ends uterine activity
(d) Generally involves blood loss of > 200 mL
(e) Involves retraction of uterine muscle

41 The following predispose to primary postpartum haemorrhage:

(a) Administration of prolonged or deep anaesthesia to the mother
(b) Twin pregnancy
(c) Oligohydramnios
(d) Prolonged labour caused by mechanical difficulty
(e) Hyperemesis gravidarum

42 Third-stage traumatic lesions:

(a) Repair of a third-degree perineal tear should not be attempted using only local anaesthesia
(b) A second-degree tear involves the perineal body and includes the anal sphincter
(c) An extensive tear of the vagina can occur without a tear in the perineum
(d) The symptoms of fistulae resulting from pressure necrosis during prolonged labour appear immediately after delivery
(e) Fistulae resulting from direct trauma should not be repaired for 2–3 months

38 (a) **False** This is a description of the passive delivery of the placenta.
   (b) **True** Intravenous syntocinon works quickly and is less likely to cause vomiting than ergometrine.
   (c) **True** There is a small risk that the contracting upper segment will close the cervix, trapping the placenta.
   (d) **False** The use of oxytocics and active management reduces the risk of postpartum haemorrhage.
   (e) **False** It begins with delivery of the anterior shoulder.

39 (a) **True** There are often decelerations due to head compression.
   (b) **True** Contractions may be stronger, but the action of pushing masks the severity of the pain.
   (c) **False** It ends with delivery of the fetus.
   (d) **False** It commences at full dilatation.
   (e) **True** The second stage may be only a few minutes in multiparae.

40 (a) **False** It starts when the fetus has been delivered.
   (b) **False** It ends when the placenta and membranes have been completely delivered.
   (c) **False** Uterine retraction continues into the puerperium.
   (d) **False** The mean blood loss is < 200 mL.
   (e) **True**

41 (a) **True** Anaesthesia, particularly the use of halothane, may cause uterine relaxation.
   (b) **True** Over-distension of the uterus predisposes to failure of retraction.
   (c) **False** Polyhydramnios, not oligohydramnios, predisposes to this because of over-distension.
   (d) **True** Inco-ordinate uterine action occurs after prolonged labour.
   (e) **False** There is no such association.

42 (a) **True** General or regional (i.e. spinal or epidural) anaesthesia should be used.
   (b) **False** Laceration of the anal sphincter places the tear in the category of the third degree.
   (c) **False** They may cause considerable bleeding and be a cause of postpartum haemorrhage.
   (d) **False** The symptoms frequently do not appear for 10 days.
   (e) **False** Recognition and immediate surgical repair constitute the correct management.

43 During vaginal breech delivery:

(a) Episiotomy should be performed immediately before delivery of the head
(b) There is a risk that a rim of cervix may retain the after-coming head
(c) Traction on the anterior groin should be used if the breech does not enter the pelvis in the second stage
(d) Lovset's manoeuvre should always be performed
(e) Pre-existing hypoxia is no more dangerous than it would be with vertex delivery

44 Obstructed labour:

(a) Always develops before full dilatation of the cervix
(b) Can usually be predicted before the onset of labour
(c) Is more common in developed countries
(d) Is inevitable in a term fetus with persistent mento-posterior position
(e) Can often be overcome by means of craniotomy if the fetus is dead

45 The following are absolute contraindications to epidural analgesia:

(a) Hypertrophic obstructive cardiomyopathy
(b) Pilonidal sinus
(c) Abruptio placentae
(d) Preterm labour
(e) Twins

46 Syntocinon augmentation of labour:

(a) Is more often required in multiparous patients
(b) Aggravates fetal distress
(c) May cause a prolonged hypertonic uterine contraction
(d) May have to be reduced as labour progresses
(e) May cause or aggravate neonatal jaundice

43 (a) **False** It should be performed when the buttock distends the perineum.
   (b) **True** This is particularly likely with a premature or footling breech.
   (c) **False** If the breech remains high, Caesarean section is indicated.
   (d) **False** This is performed for nuchal displacement of the arms.
   (e) **False** A degree of asphyxia is inevitable in vaginal breech delivery because the cord is obstructed once the chest enters the pelvis. This can only be tolerated if the fetus is well oxygenated prior to delivery.

44 (a) **False** In some cases, labour proceeds to full dilatation, and the fetal head is then unable to descend through the pelvis.
   (b) **False** Prediction is rarely possible (e.g. cases with a bony deformity of the pelvis).
   (c) **False** The mean pelvic size is smaller in non-developed countries.
   (d) **True** Delivery is only possible if rotation to the mento-anterior position occurs.
   (e) **True** Craniotomy will be effective if the fetus is presenting by the vertex; more complex destructive operations or Caesarean section are required for an impacted, dead transverse lie.

45 (a) **True** In this condition, any reduction in end diastolic volume narrows the ventricular outflow tract and aggravates failure.
   (b) **True** Any local sepsis will predispose to an epidural abscess.
   (c) **True** Shock is likely to be aggravated by abolishing protective vasoconstruction.
   (d) **False** By avoiding the use of drugs which inhibit respiration, this technique may be especially suitable for premature labour.
   (e) **False** Epidural analgesia is suitable for twin delivery and may even be beneficial

46 (a) **False** Hypotonic inertia is more common in primiparous women.
   (b) **True** Uterine contractions always obstruct placental blood flow. They become stronger with syntocinon, and the recovery phase between contractions is shortened.
   (c) **True** This causes fetal distress, and may cause uterine rupture.
   (d) **True** Labour is a self-perpetuating process, and the dose may have to be reduced if contractions occur too frequently.
   (e) **True** This may be due in part to the antidiuretic effect of oxytocin causing red cells to swell and become less distensible. Such cells are more rapidly removed from the circulation.

LABOUR

47 Fetal hypoxaemia during the first stage of labour:

(a) Always causes type II dips (late decelerations)
(b) Can be diagnosed with a high degree of confidence if meconium is present
(c) Is associated with an accumulation of lactic acid in the fetus
(d) Should be treated with an infusion of bicarbonate
(e) Can be helped by oxygen and glucose in the short term, while making preparations for Caesarean section

48 The following predispose to fetal hypoxaemia in labour:

(a) The supine position
(b) Pre-eclampsia
(c) Renal disease
(d) Lupus erythematosus
(e) Pethidine administration

49 Prior to engagement of the fetal head:

(a) The head usually enters the pelvis in an occipito-transverse position
(b) A trial of forceps may be carried out provided that the vertex has passed the plane of the pelvic inlet
(c) Three-fifths or more of the head are palpable abdominally
(d) Induction of labour should not be performed
(e) Spontaneous labour is unlikely to start

50 Prolapse of the umbilical cord:

(a) May occur while the membranes are still intact
(b) Is a risk of induction of labour with prostaglandin pessaries
(c) Has an incidence of 1% of labours
(d) Is more common in singleton than in twin deliveries
(e) Causes severe respiratory acidosis in the fetus

47 (a) **False** Although type II dips are often caused by fetal hypoxaemia, other cardiotocograph changes (e.g. bradycardia, loss of short-term variation) may also occur.

(b) **False** The passage of meconium due to vagal stimulation and contraction of the bowel may occur in fetal hypoxaemia, but the association is not strong.

(c) **True** Fetal hypoxaemia causes anaerobic metabolism and lactate accumulation.

(d) **False** Although the fetus is acidotic, bicarbonate is not helpful as it does not cross the placenta well.

(e) **False** Oxygen is of benefit, but glucose compounds lactate accumulation in the fetus.

48 (a) **True** Pressure on the inferior vena cava diminishes venous return to the right side of the heart, causing hypotension and reduced placental blood flow.

(b) **True** Narrowing of the spiral arteries and vasospasm reduce placental blood flow.

(c) **True**

(d) **True** Patients with the lupus anticoagulant develop placental microthrombi.

(e) **False** This predisposes to poor respiratory effort after delivery.

49 (a) **True** This is the usual position at engagement.

(b) **False** This may still be a high head. As such, a trial of forceps is inadvisable.

(c) **True**

(d) **False** Provided that the head is stably over the brim of the pelvis, induction with prostaglandins may be attempted.

(e) **False** In 60% of multiparous cases and 40% of primiparous cases, the head does not engage prior to labour.

50 (a) **False** In an intact bag of membranes, this is a cord presentation.

(b) **False** It is a risk of artificial rupture of membranes with a high presenting part.

(c) **False** A more accurate figure would be 0.3%.

(d) **False** It is very common with the second twin, especially if the membranes rupture before contractions resume or the presenting part descends.

(e) **True** This is the initial effect of rapidly accumulating carbon dioxide. Later the hypoxia will lead to a superimposed metabolic acidosis.

51 The occipito-posterior position:

  (a) Is an example of a malpresentation

  (b) Usually turns to deliver as the occipito-anterior position

  (c) May proceed to deep transverse arrest

  (d) Is associated with a prolonged first stage

  (e) Is associated with a prolonged second stage

51 (a) **False** It is a malposition. Breech and face are malpresentations.
 (b) **True** This happens in about 80% of cases.
 (c) **True** This occurs when rotation of the occiput is arrested in the transverse position.
 (d) **True** The head tends to be deflexed in the sub-occipito frontal (10 cm) diameter.
 (e) **True** Rotation takes place in the late first and second stages.

THE PUERPERIUM

52 After delivery:

(a) A vulvovaginal haematoma should not be incised for fear of causing an abscess

(b) Third-degree tear usually leads to rectal incontinence despite immediate suture

(c) Bimanual compression is useful for expelling a retained placenta

(d) A much more concentrated oxytocin infusion may be used than when in labour

(e) Maternal pyrexia may be a physiological occurrence

53 The following organisms are recognized causes of puerperal pelvic sepsis:

(a) *Escherichia coli*

(b) Haemolytic streptoccocus (group A)

(c) *Haemophilus influenzae*

(d) *Clostridium welchii*

(e) *Staphylococcus aureus*

54 Puerperal sepsis due to haemolytic *Streptococcus* (group A):

(a) May cause rigors

(b) Is the commonest cause of maternal mortality

(c) Is likely to be caused by endogenous infection

(d) Haemoglobinuria is usual

(e) Is treated with tetracycline

55 Breastfeeding has the following advantages over bottle-feeding:

(a) Human milk contains more protein

(b) Human milk contains more carbohydrate

(c) There is a lower incidence of cot death in breastfed infants

(d) There is a lower incidence of atopic conditions in breastfed infants

(e) It needs to be given less frequently

52 (a) **False** If tense, painful or enlarging, it is best to decompress it and ligate the bleeding vessel.
   (b) **False** The prognosis is excellent with adequate repair.
   (c) **False** A retained placenta should be removed manually. Bimanual compression is useful for atonic postpartum haemorrhage.
   (d) **True** In the treatment of atonic postpartum haemorrhage, doses such as 50 units in 500 mL may be given at a rate of 30–60 drops/minute without the risk of uterine rupture.
   (e) **False** A maternal pyrexia should be treated seriously.

53 (a) **True** This is an endogenous organism and a common cause of local perineal infection.
   (b) **True** This is an exogenous organism and a cause of severe infection.
   (c) **False**
   (d) **True** Clostridial infection is extremely rare, but it may occur with extensive tissue damage.
   (e) **True** *Staphylococcus aureus* is an increasing problem, due to the development of resistant strains.

54 (a) **True** It is not infrequently associated with rigors.
   (b) **False** It is now an infrequent cause of maternal mortality in the UK.
   (c) **False** The source of infection is likely to be from attendants.
   (d) **False** This occurs in clostridial infection.
   (e) **False** Penicillin is the treatment of choice.

55 (a) **False** There is too much protein in cow's milk.
   (b) **True**
   (c) **True** However, cause and effect are unproven.
   (d) **True** Cow's milk protein provides a powerful antigenic stimulus.
   (e) **False** Bottle feeds may be given less frequently because larger volumes can be given.

56 Engorgement of the breasts in a lactating mother is treated by:

(a) Stopping feeding for 24 hours
(b) Giving diuretics
(c) Manual or mechanical expression
(d) Discarding brassières
(e) Analgesics

57 In puerperal breast abscess:

(a) Streptococci are the commonest infecting organisms
(b) Suppression of lactation is advisable
(c) Surgical drainage is rarely necessary
(d) The whole breast is affected
(e) Antibiotics should always be given

56 (a) **False** Encouragement of the flow is important.
  (b) **False** Diuretics are potentially harmful to the baby.
  (c) **True** This may be the only way to relieve the discomfort.
  (d) **False** Firm support is important.
  (e) **True**

57 (a) **False** *Staphylococcus aureus* is the commonest organism.
  (b) **True** In mastitis, temporary suspension of breastfeeding may suffice, but if there is an abscess, cessation of lactation is invariably necessary.
  (c) **False** It is always necessary once an abscess has occurred.
  (d) **False** It is usually segmental.
  (e) **True**

PRE-ECLAMPSIA AND GROWTH RESTRICTION

58 Small-for-dates babies are particularly liable to develop:

(a) Hypoglycaemia
(b) Hypothermia
(c) Respiratory distress syndrome (RDS)
(d) Anaemia
(e) Pneumonia

59 In eclampsia:

(a) Large doses of intravenous sedation are given
(b) Caesarean section must be performed whether the fetus is dead or alive
(c) Hypotensive drugs should not be used
(d) Ergometrine should be avoided in the third stage of labour
(e) Urinary output is increased

60 In pre-eclamptic toxaemia:

(a) There is an increase in extracellular sodium
(b) Proteinurea is the earliest sign
(c) Serum uric acid levels tend to decrease
(d) The hepatic lesion shows patchy haemorrhage and necrosis
(e) There is disturbance of the clotting mechanism

61 There is an increased risk of developing pre-eclampsia with:

(a) Increasing maternal age
(b) High parity
(c) Hydatidiform mole
(d) Maternal cardiac disease
(e) Diabetes

58 (a) **True** Because depletion of glycogen stores has occurred *in utero*.
  (b) **True** Because the lack of subcutaneous fat impairs heat conservation.
  (c) **False** Pre-term babies, not small-for-dates babies, develop RDS.
  (d) **False** Pre-term babies are susceptible to anaemia.
  (e) **False** Small-for-dates babies are not particularly prone to infection.

59 (a) **True** Magnesium sulphate infusion is increasingly accepted as the sedative of choice.
  (b) **False** If the fetus is dead or the cervix is favourable, induction of labour may be attempted.
  (c) **False** Hypotensives are used to reduce the risk of cerebral haemorrhage.
  (d) **True** The vasoconstrictor effect raises the blood pressure; syntocinon is preferable.
  (e) **False** There is oliguria, which may progress to renal failure.

60 (a) **True** There is retention of both water and sodium.
  (b) **False** Weight gain, oedema and hypertension usually precede proteinurea.
  (c) **False** Levels increase as a result of an alteration in renal tubular function.
  (d) **True** Characteristic red and yellow focal areas are seen.
  (e) **True** There is a fall in the number of platelets, and an increase in the level of fibrin degradation products.

61 (a) **True** It is more common in women over 35 years of age.
  (b) **False** It is more common in primagravid women.
  (c) **True** The hypertension is severe and it often starts as early as 16–20 weeks.
  (d) **False** There is no relationship with cardiac disease.
  (e) **True** This is assumed to be due to diabetic vascular disease.

62 Impaired fetal growth:

(a) Is symmetrical if the fetal head and abdomen are equally reduced in size
(b) Has long-term effects on postnatal growth if it is asymmetrical in type
(c) Is rarely associated with hypoxia and acidosis if it is symmetrical in type
(d) May be due to maternal heroin abuse if it is asymmetrical in type
(e) May be assessed with a single ultrasound examination in the third trimester

63 Antenatal management of an asymmetrically small fetus should include:

(a) Ultrasound examination to measure growth
(b) Maternal scoring of fetal movements
(c) Serial measurement of plasma oestradiol or human placental lactogen (HPL)
(d) Cardiotocography
(e) Fetal scalp sampling

62 (a) **True** All parts of fetal growth velocity are affected equally.
   (b) **False** This reflects an inadequate supply of nutrients. Postnatal catch-up growth will occur.
   (c) **True** It is more likely to be constitutional or due to a specific problem (aneuploidy).
   (d) **True** Heroin abuse, alcohol consumption and smoking all cause asymmetrical growth impairment.
   (e) **False** Serial ultrasound measurements are necessary to confirm impaired fetal growth.

63 (a) **True** A fall-off in growth rate may prompt delivery.
   (b) **True** A reduction in fetal movements may indicate fetal hypoxia.
   (c) **False** Placental hormones are now known to be an insensitive test of fetal well-being.
   (d) **True** This is the most popular method of fetal assessment.
   (e) **False** This can only be done in labour.

PRE-ECLAMPSIA AND GROWTH RESTRICTION

PRENATAL DIAGNOSIS

64 The following statements are true of tests used in prenatal diagnosis:

(a) Serum biochemistry is superior to maternal age as a screening test for Down's syndrome

(b) Maternal serum alpha-fetoprotein is a diagnostic test for neural-tube defects

(c) Chorionic villus sampling (CVS) has a lower pregnancy loss rate than amniocentesis

(d) Tests using DNA technology can be performed on amniocentesis specimens

(e) Chorionic villus sampling can only be performed before 12 weeks' gestation

65 Biochemical screening for chromosomal abnormalities:

(a) Can provide risk estimates for trisomy 18

(b) Includes hCG, low levels of which are associated with Down's syndrome

(c) Is most accurate when femur length is used to assess gestational age

(d) Can be an indicator of other poor fetal outcomes

(e) Does not take maternal age into account

66 Congenital abnormality:

(a) Cystic fibrosis is a congenital abnormality, while Huntington's chorea is not

(b) Down's syndrome is more common than congenital heart defects

(c) Trisomies 13, 18 and 21 are equally common at conception

(d) The prevalence of sex chromosome abnormalities does not depend on maternal age

(e) Fragile X syndrome can be inherited from a mentally normal 'carrier' father

67 Neural-tube defects:

(a) Occur because of a poor preconceptual maternal diet

(b) The majority of these defects occur at the cranial end of the spine

(c) The prognosis for spina bifida depends on the spinal level of the lesion

(d) With a previous affected sibling, the recurrence risk is 1%

(e) A supplement of 400µg folic acid daily significantly reduces the risk of recurrence

64 (a) **True** Biochemical screening has a sensitivity of 60–70%, compared to 30–40% for maternal age.
   (b) **False** It is a *screening* test, requiring confirmation by ultrasound.
   (c) **False** A 16-week amniocentesis has the same procedure-related loss rate as CVS.
   (d) **True** The larger amounts of DNA in CVS make this the preferred method of sampling.
   (e) **False** It is usually performed between 8 and 20 weeks, but the risk of fetal damage is increased before 10 weeks.

65 (a) **True** Although the test is designed for screening for Down's syndrome, a low level of HCG is a marker for trisomy 18.
   (b) **False** hCG levels are raised in Down's syndrome.
   (c) **False** Femur length is shorter in Down's fetuses, thus reducing the sensitivity of the test.
   (d) **True** Elevated alpha-fetoprotein levels indicate increased risk of neural-tube defects and placental dysfunction.
   (e) **False** Maternal age and weight are included in the risk calculation.

66 (a) **False** 'Congenital' means conferred by birth, regardless of the age of onset.
   (b) **False** The prevalence of Down's syndrome (1.5/1000) is less than that of heart defects (8/1000).
   (c) **True** The intrauterine lethality (90–95%) of trisomy 13/18 reduces their prevalence at birth.
   (d) **True** Autosomal, not sex chromosome, abnormalities increase with advancing maternal age.
   (e) **True** The fragile X gene may hypermethylate/form multiple repeats in affected male offspring of a normal male parent.

67 (a) **False** There are environmental, genetic, pharmacological and geographical aetiologies.
   (b) **True** Around 70–80% of neural-tube defects are anencephaly or encephaloceles.
   (c) **True** The spinal level and number of segments involved determine the prognosis.
   (d) **False** The recurrence risk will be as high as 5%.
   (e) **False** A daily supplement of 4mg is required to reduce the recurrence

MULTIPLE PREGNANCY

68 The incidence of multiple pregnancy is increased:

(a) In Afro-Caribbeans
(b) In women treated with bromocriptine for infertility
(c) In women treated by *in vitro* fertilization
(d) With advancing maternal age
(e) In first pregnancies

69 In twin delivery:

(a) The first twin is at greater risk than the second
(b) Labour usually occurs before term
(c) Epidural analgesia is best avoided
(d) There is an increased risk of postpartum haemorrhage
(e) The commonest presentation is one cephalic, one breech

70 Twin zygosity and chorionicity:

(a) Chorionicity is determined by ultrasound, while zygosity usually requires DNA testing
(b) Chorionicity does not affect pregnancy outcome
(c) Placental insufficiency occurs more frequently in twins than in singletons
(d) Congenital abnormalities are twice as likely in monochorionic twins as in dichorionic twins
(e) Twin–twin transfusion syndrome (TTTS) can occur in diamniotic twins

68 (a) **True** In some West African tribes the incidence is 1 in 30 (cf. 1 in 90 in Caucasians).

   (b) **False** Bromocriptine does not induce multiple ovulation.

   (c) **True** The replacement of several embryos leads to a greater risk of multiple pregnancy.

   (d) **True** Binovular twinning increases with age up to about 40 years.

   (e) **False** It is commonest in multigravid women.

69 (a) **False** Fetal mortality and morbidity are greater in the second twin.

   (b) **True** Over-distension of the uterus leads to pre-term labour.

   (c) **False** Epidural analgesia is ideal, in preparation for any second-stage difficulties.

   (d) **True** The larger placental site and uterine over-distension are aetiological factors.

   (e) **False** The commonest presentation is cephalic–cephalic (45% of cases).

70 (a) **True** Chorionicity is determined from the number of placentas and membrane characteristics.

   (b) **False** Perinatal mortality is significantly higher in monochorionic pregnancies.

   (c) **True** Approximately 25% of twins will develop a significant growth discrepancy.

   (d) **True** Congenital abnormality is also twice as likely in dichorionic twins compared to singletons.

   (e) **True** TTTS can only occur in monochorionic twins, regardless of amnionicity.

ANTENATAL OBSTETRIC COMPLICATIONS

71 Coagulation failure is an important common complication of:

(a) Placenta praevia
(b) Abruptio placentae
(c) Amniotic fluid embolus
(d) Gram-negative septicaemia
(e) Uterine rupture

72 The following may cause intrauterine death of the fetus:

(a) Diabetes mellitus
(b) Respiratory distress syndrome (RDS)
(c) Hydrops fetalis
(d) A sudden emotional shock to the mother
(e) Syphilis

73 In cases of intrauterine death:

(a) Induction of labour should always begin immediately
(b) It is always best to give the parents immediate, detailed information about the possible cause
(c) The baby must always be shown to the parents
(d) It is important to discuss contraception prior to hospital discharge
(e) Lactation is likely to occur and become distressing

74 When intrauterine death of the fetus occurs in the third trimester:

(a) Caesarean section should be performed to deliver the fetus
(b) There is a tendency to thromboembolism
(c) There is a danger of anaerobic infection
(d) Lactation will not occur after delivery
(e) The birth of the baby must be registered

75 Polyhydramnios is associated with the following:

(a) Chorioangioma of the placenta
(b) Maternal diabetes
(c) Hydatidiform mole
(d) Hydrops fetalis
(e) Intrauterine growth retardation of the fetus

71 (a) **False** There is straightforward haemorrhage in this condition.
  (b) **True** Disseminated intravascular coagulation is thought to occur as a result of thromboplastin release from the placental site.
  (c) **True** There is widespread disseminated intravascular coagulation.
  (d) **True** Endotoxins, kinins and complement stimulate the clotting mechanism.
  (e) **False** Although uterine rupture may lead to shock and collapse, disseminated intravascular coagulation does not usually occur.

72 (a) **True** Poorly controlled diabetes may lead to sudden fetal death.
  (b) **False** This is a cause of neonatal death.
  (c) **True** Hydrops fetalis, whatever the cause, may lead to fetal death.
  (d) **False** This only occurs in fiction.
  (e) **True** Untreated syphilis is one of the rare causes.

73 (a) **False** Unless there are good medical reasons, parents can be given time to take in the news.
  (b) **False** Parents are shocked and unable to take in detailed information immediately.
  (c) **False** This should be offered, but some parents will not want to see the baby.
  (d) **True** This is difficult and often forgotten, but it should be discussed.
  (e) **True** The mother needs to be warned of this and offered suppression of lactation.

74 (a) **False** Vaginal delivery is far preferable.
  (b) **False** Hypofibrinogenaemia may occur, resulting in failure of blood coagulation.
  (c) **True** After membrane rupture, there is an ideal culture medium for anaerobic organisms.
  (d) **False** Suppression of lactation should be considered.
  (e) **True** It must be registered as a stillbirth.

75 (a) **True** This is a rare fetal cause.
  (b) **True** This is likely if the diabetes is poorly controlled, and it is due to fetal polyuria.
  (c) **False** The uterus is filled with molar tissue.
  (d) **True** This is often the case in severe rhesus iso-immunization.
  (e) **False** It is often associated with oligohydramnios.

76 Oligohydramnios is associated with the following fetal conditions:

(a) Tracheo-oesophageal fistula
(b) Talipes
(c) Potter's syndrome
(d) Intrauterine growth retardation
(e) Anencephaly

77 Antepartum haemorrhage:

(a) Is defined as bleeding from the genital tract in pregnancy
(b) May be complicated by hypofibrinogenaemia
(c) Requires assessment by vaginal examination
(d) May be caused by cervical carcinoma
(e) Is always painless

78 To prevent rhesus disease iso-immunization anti-D should be given to rhesus-negative women:

(a) Within 72 hours of delivery of a rhesus-positive child
(b) Who are known to have rhesus antibodies, within 72 hours of delivery
(c) Following a termination of pregnancy, even when the father is known to be heterozygous
(d) When an external cephalic version has been performed
(e) Following a small (< 30 mL) antepartum haemorrhage

79 In rhesus iso-immunization the following tests may be helpful:

(a) Rhesus antibody titre in liquor
(b) Liquor bilirubin level
(c) Maternal serum bilirubin
(d) Direct Coombs' test on cord blood
(e) Rhesus genotype of father

76 (a) **False** This causes polyhydramnios due to failure of swallowing.
　　(b) **True** Limb deformations occur because of local pressure.
　　(c) **True** Renal agenesis results in lack of liquor.
　　(d) **True** Poor placental function is associated with oligohydramnios.
　　(e) **False** This is often associated with polyhydramnios due to inability of the fetus to swallow.

77 (a) **False** It is bleeding from the genital tract after fetal viability (*c*. 24 weeks).
　　(b) **True** This occurs in placental abruption, which is one cause of antepartum haemorrhage.
　　(c) **False** Vaginal examination is dangerous until placenta praevia has been ruled out.
　　(d) **True** This is an incidental cause of antepartum haemorrhage.
　　(e) **False** Placental abruption is usually painful, whilst bleeding from placenta praevia is painless.

78 (a) **True** This will prevent iso-immunization.
　　(b) **False** Giving anti-D once there are rhesus antibodies is a useless exercise.
　　(c) **True** A heterozygous father has a 50% chance of producing a rhesus-positive offspring.
　　(d) **True** The trauma of version may produce feto-maternal haemorrhage.
　　(e) **True** Any amount of antepartum haemorrhage may cause rhesus iso-immunization.

79 (a) **False** Rhesus antibody titre in *maternal blood* is performed routinely and may be useful.
　　(b) **True** This is measured spectrophotometrically on liquor obtained at an amniocentesis.
　　(c) **False** The maternal bilirubin level is not altered in rhesus iso-immunization.
　　(d) **True** This test confirms whether the baby is affected.
　　(e) **True** If the partner is heterozygous, there is a 50% chance that the baby will be unaffected.

80 The following predispose to deep venous thrombosis:

  (a) Caesarean section
  (b) Antenatal bed rest
  (c) Breastfeeding
  (d) Varicose veins
  (e) Pelvic infection

81 Venous thromboembolism:

  (a) Is the commonest cause of maternal death in the world
  (b) Pregnancy results in an imbalance between the thrombolytic and fibrinolytic systems
  (c) Caused by thrombophilia may be associated with recurrent miscarriage
  (d) Pregnant women with calf pain should have thromboprophylaxis until it is investigated
  (e) Heparin can be given indefinitely, as it does not cross the placenta

80 (a) **True** Abdominal delivery considerably increases the risk of thrombo-embolism.

(b) **True** If other risk factors are present (e.g. age, obesity), anticoagulants should be considered.

(c) **False** Suppression of lactation with oestrogen predisposes to thrombosis.

(d) **False** Varicose veins increase the risk of *superficial* thrombophlebitis.

(e) **True** This applies to postpartum infection in maternity patients.

81 (a) **False** It is the commonest cause of maternal death in the UK.

(b) **True** Pregnancy is a hypercoagulable state.

(c) **True** Thrombophilias include protein S, protein C and antithrombin III deficiency .

(d) **True** Heparin can be stopped if venography or Doppler refutes the diagnosis of deep venous thrombosis.

(e) **False** It does not cross the placenta, but long-term therapy causes bone demineralization.

ANTENATAL OBSTETRIC COMPLICATIONS

PERINATAL INFECTIONS

82 The following may cause congenital infection of the fetus:

    (a) Cytomegalovirus
    (b) Varicella
    (c) Hepatitis B
    (d) Herpes
    (e) Parvovirus

83 With regard to HIV testing in pregnancy:

    (a) The antibody test may take 1 month to become positive after exposure
    (b) The time to development of AIDS is 10 years without treatment
    (c) The vertical transmission rate is approximately 15%
    (d) With intervention, the vertical transmission rate can be reduced to 3%
    (e) Stopping breastfeeding is the most effective way to prevent vertical transmission

84 Herpes infection in pregnancy:

    (a) If infection occurs in the first trimester, termination of pregnancy should be offered in view of the risk of congenital infection.
    (b) Topical acyclovir is effective in the treatment of genital herpes
    (c) Neonatal infection has a mortality of 50%
    (d) Caesarean section is recommended if there is evidence of active primary herpes in labour
    (e) Caesarean section is recommended if there is evidence of active secondary herpes in labour

82 (a) **True** It causes microcephaly, blindness and developmental delay.
   (b) **True** It may cause hypoplastic limbs, skin scarring and CNS abnormalities.
   (c) **False** It may cause neonatal infection.
   (d) **True** There is a rare syndrome that causes micro-ophthalmia and microcephaly.
   (e) **True** It can cause fetal pancytopenia and hydrops.

83 (a) **False** The test may take 3 months to become reactive.
   (b) **True** It is possible to remain healthy for 15 years with treatment.
   (c) **False** Vertical transmission occurs in 25–40% of pregnancies.
   (d) **True** These interventions include anti-retroviral drugs, Caesarean section and avoidance of breastfeeding.
   (e) **True** About 15% of vertical transmission is thought to be due to breastfeeding.

84 (a) **False** Congenital abnormality is very rare with herpes infection.
   (b) **False**
   (c) **False** Mortality is 70%, and is reduced to 40% with neonatal intravenous acyclovir.
   (d) **True** Unless membranes have been ruptured for longer than 4 hours.
   (e) **False** Regardless of membrane rupture.

MEDICAL DISEASES COMPLICATING PREGNANCY

85 The following are correct associations:

    (a) Anencephaly and face presentation
    (b) Advancing maternal age and Turner's syndrome
    (c) Hydatidiform mole and pre-eclampsia
    (d) Diabetes mellitus and neonatal hyperglycaemia
    (e) Precipitate labour and postpartum haemorrhage

86 Hyperthyroidism in pregnancy:

    (a) Should be treated surgically rather than with carbimazole
    (b) May lead to neonatal hyperthyroidism even though the mother's disease is treated
    (c) Should not be treated with anti-thyroid drugs
    (d) Can be diagnosed by total T_4 measurement
    (e) Is always associated with increased long-acting thyroid stimulator

87 In sickle-cell disorders:

    (a) There is failure of formation of the beta-chain of haemoglobin
    (b) The haemoglobin level rarely falls below 9.0 g/dL
    (c) There is a high incidence in Afro-Caribbeans and Asians
    (d) Iron deficiency is usual
    (e) Crisis is unlikely to occur with the trait

88 Diabetes mellitus in pregnancy is associated with the following:

    (a) Increased incidence of congenital defects
    (b) Increased insulin requirements
    (c) Increased risk of placental abruption
    (d) A high incidence of vaginal *Trichomonas* infection
    (e) Fetal macrosomia

85 (a) **True** The abnormal head faces downwards, making face presentation more likely.

  (b) **False** Unlike trisomies, Turner's syndrome is not dependent on maternal age.

  (c) **True** In this condition, pre-eclampsia occurs early in pregnancy (at 16–20 weeks).

  (d) **False** Hypoglycaemia is a problem because of fetal hyperinsulinaemia.

  (e) **True** This usually occurs in a grand multiparous patient and there is uterine atony.

86 (a) **False** It is usually treated medically until the postnatal thyroid surgery.

  (b) **True** Because long-acting thyroid-stimulating hormone may cross the placenta.

  (c) **False** Although these drugs cross the placenta, they rarely affect fetal thyroid function.

  (d) **False** Total T_4 levels are normally raised in pregnancy. Free thyroxine levels are required.

  (e) **False** Long-acting thyroid stimulator is only rarely present.

87 (a) **False** Rather than failure, there is an alteration in the amino-acid structure of the chain.

  (b) **False** Severe anaemia may occur in sickle-cell disease.

  (c) **False** There is a high incidence in Afro-Caribbeans, but not in Asians.

  (d) **False** Iron stores are usually adequate.

  (e) **True** The concentration of haemoglobin S is usually too low for sickling to occur.

88 (a) **True** The risk of congenital abnormality is related to the degree of pre-conceptual control.

  (b) **True** The insulin requirements frequently double.

  (c) **False** Although the placenta is larger, there is no increased risk of abruption.

  (d) **False** It is vaginal *Candida* infection which is associated with diabetes.

  (e) **True** Poorly controlled diabetes leads to fetal macrosomia and risk of obstructed labour.

89 In acute pyelonephritis in pregnancy:

   (a) The left kidney is affected more often than the right
   (b) The temperature rarely exceeds 39°C
   (c) Antibiotics should be started before bacteriological results are available
   (d) The incidence of fetal growth retardation and preterm labour is increased
   (e) Intravenous pyelography should be performed promptly

90 In cardiac disease in pregnancy:

   (a) Congenital heart disease is the commonest cause
   (b) Cardiac failure should not be treated with digoxin
   (c) Delivery should be by planned Caesarean section
   (d) Cardiac surgery is absolutely contraindicated
   (e) Ergometrine should be avoided in the third stage

91 The following drugs are known to be teratogenic:

   (a) Phenobarbitone
   (b) Diazepam
   (c) Alpha-methyldopa
   (d) Erythromycin
   (e) Thiazide diuretics

92 The following conditions are usually exacerbated during pregnancy:

   (a) Peptic ulcer
   (b) Multiple sclerosis
   (c) Neuralgia parasthetica
   (d) Dental caries
   (e) Psoriasis

89 (a) **False** The right kidney is affected more often than the left.
   (b) **False** Fevers of 39.5°C and above are common, and are often associated with rigors.
   (c) **True** Treatment is started promptly because of the risk of septicaemia and preterm labour.
   (d) **True** Fetal growth retardation is more likely if there is chronic renal disease.
   (e) **False** This treatment is only indicated for recurrent attacks of pyelonephritis (usually performed postnatally).

90 (a) **True** Today, rheumatic heart disease causes less than 50% of valvular abnormalities.
   (b) **False** Digoxin is perfectly safe in pregnancy.
   (c) **False** Caesarean section is only advised for obstetric reasons.
   (d) **False** Cardiopulmonary bypass and open-heart surgery carries a considerable risk of fetal loss, but closed heart surgery may be performed with reasonable safety.
   (e) **True** Ergometrine, by causing an increase in blood pressure, may precipitate cardiac failure.

91 (a) **False** Phenytoin, usually given with phenobarbitone, may cause chondrodysplasia punctata.
   (b) **False** Diazepam may cause cardiac and respiratory depression, but is not teratogenic.
   (c) **False** This drug and beta-blockers are the most widely used treatments for hypertension in pregnancy.
   (d) **False** Erythromycin, penicillin and cephalosporins are safe in pregnancy. Sulphonamides may aggravate neonatal jaundice, tetracyclines damage teeth and bones, aminoglycosides occasionally damage the VIIIth nerve and trimethoprim antagonizes folate and therefore constitutes a theoretical teratogenic risk.
   (e) **False** However, they may aggravate neonatal thrombocytopenia.

92 (a) **False** Gastric acidity is often reduced, but reflux oesophagitis is more common.
   (b) **False** Relapse may occur after delivery.
   (c) **True** This condition is caused by entrapment of the lateral cutaneous nerve of the thigh.
   (d) **True** Gingivitis is common in pregnancy, and this exacerbates dental caries.
   (e) **False** The increase in cortisol levels often improves psoriasis.

MEDICAL DISEASES COMPLICATING PREGNANCY

93 Cholestasis in pregnancy:

(a) Characteristically presents with pruritus and a maculo-papular rash
(b) Presents in the mid second trimester
(c) Is treated by the use of ursodeoxycholic acid (UDCA)
(d) Delivery is normally indicated at 38 weeks in view of the fetal risks
(e) Maternal oral vitamin K is usually prescribed

93 (a) **False** There is no rash in cholestasis (except excoriation).
   (b) **False** It usually presents in the late third trimester.
   (c) **False** UDCA provides symptomatic relief only. Fetal risks remain unaltered.
   (d) **True** In view of the risk of unexplained stillbirth.
   (e) **True** Vitamin K is thought to reduce the risk of postpartum haemorrhage.

MEDICAL DISEASES COMPLICATING PREGNANCY

SECOND-TRIMESTER MISCARRIAGE AND PRETERM LABOUR

94 Second-trimester miscarriage:

(a) Is typically painless
(b) Occurs between 12 and 24 weeks' gestation
(c) Can be associated with rupture of membranes
(d) Is diagnosed after exclusion of infection, haemorrhage and multiple pregnancy
(e) Antibiotic prophylaxis is usually given

95 Spontaneous preterm labour:

(a) Multiple pregnancy is the commonest cause
(b) Is defined as labour before week 34
(c) Does not tend to recur in subsequent pregnancies
(d) Is the commonest cause of perinatal mortality
(e) Is common in pre-eclampsia

96 The following are contraindications to intravenous beta-adrenergic stimulant therapy:

(a) Preterm labour
(b) Fetal distress in labour
(c) Previous Caesarean section
(d) Asthma
(e) Insulin-dependent diabetes

94 (a) **False** Backache, contractions and vaginal bleeding are typical.
   (b) **True** After 24 weeks, the same symptoms/signs would be termed preterm labour.
   (c) **True** Rupture of membranes may be the presenting symptom.
   (d) **False** These are presumed aetiological factors.
   (e) **False** Antibiotics are only used if there is strong evidence of infection.

95 (a) **False** Unexplained/idiopathic causes are by far the most common.
   (b) **False** It is defined as labour before week 37.
   (c) **False** A previous history of premature delivery is a risk factor for another preterm delivery.
   (d) **True**
   (e) **False** However, early labour is often induced for this reason.

96 (a) **False** This is the primary indication for this therapy.
   (b) **False** This therapy may be useful in certain situations (e.g. hyperstimulation).
   (c) **False**
   (d) **False** This is an indication for beta-adrenergic stimulant therapy. Cardiac disease, especially aortic and mitral stenosis, is a contraindication.
   (e) **True** The insulin requirement increases about five-fold on this treatment.

OPERATIVE INTERVENTION IN OBSTETRICS

97 The following are always indications for Caesarean section:

   (a) Hydrocephalus

   (b) Type 4 placenta praevia (major praevia)

   (c) Abruptio placentae

   (d) Untreated stage Ib cancer of the cervix

   (e) Active primary genital herpes

98 Episiotomy:

   (a) Allows widening of the birth canal

   (b) Can be midline or mediolateral in site

   (c) If midline bleeds less, is easier to repair and heals more quickly

   (d) Must be performed for shoulder dystocia and instrumental delivery

   (e) Involvement of the anal sphincter is classified as third/fourth degree

99 Instrumental vaginal delivery:

   (a) The only prerequisite is full cervical dilatation

   (b) Forceps may be used if the ventouse fails

   (c) Ventouse cannot be used for preterm deliveries (< 34 weeks)

   (d) Forceps are used in breech delivery

   (e) Ventouse cannot be used for rotational (occipito-transverse/posterior) deliveries

97 (a) **False** Fetuses with hydrocephalus can usually be delivered vaginally with or without decompression (transcervically or transabdominally).
   (b) **True** This is the safest method of delivery, even if the fetus is dead.
   (c) **False** Vaginal delivery is preferable, unless the fetus or the mother become compromised.
   (d) **True** Cervical dilatation and vaginal delivery are thought to disseminate cancer cells.
   (e) **True** Vaginal delivery increases the risk of congenital herpes encephalitis, unless more than 4 hours have elapsed since rupture of the membranes.

98 (a) **False** Episiotomy widens the vulval outlet only.
   (b) **True** Mediolateral episiotomies are preferred in the UK.
   (c) **True** However, it is more likely to extend to involve the anal sphincter.
   (d) **False** These are relative indications only.
   (e) **True**

99 (a) **False** Adequate analgesia, an engaged head and an empty bladder are required.
   (b) **False** This is not recommended practice.
   (c) **True** There is an increased incidence of cranial trauma with this method.
   (d) **True** They are used to deliver the after-coming head in a controlled manner.
   (e) **False** Selection of an appropriate cup permits rotational deliveries with the ventouse.

OBSTETRIC EMERGENCIES

100 Postpartum haemorrhage:

   (a) Is defined as a blood loss of 1 L

   (b) Is less likely if oxytocics are administered routinely in the third stage of labour

   (c) Is primary if it occurs within the first 12 hours

   (d) Is common after both placenta praevia and abruptio placentae

   (e) May require manual removal of the placenta

101 Eclampsia:

   (a) Is proteinuric hypertension in pregnancy associated with tissue oedema

   (b) Is preceded by a poorly characterized 'fulminant' phase

   (c) Has a mortality of 2%

   (d) Is due to a cerebrovascular event

   (e) The treatment of choice is magnesium sulphate

102 Pulmonary embolism (PE):

   (a) Is the leading cause of maternal mortality in the world

   (b) Presents with chest pain, breathlessness and haemoptysis

   (c) May be managed conservatively

   (d) One differential diagnosis for PE is amniotic fluid embolism

   (e) PEs are more common in the antenatal period

OBSTETRIC EMERGENCIES

100 (a) **False** Blood loss of > 500 mL is the definition.
　　(b) **True** This has been confirmed by several randomized trials.
　　(c) **False** Secondary postpartum haemorrhage occurs after 24 hours.
　　(d) **True** This is due to poor contraction of the placental bed and consumptive coagulopathy.
　　(e) **True** If bleeding continues and the placenta remains undelivered.

101 (a) **False** It is a *grand mal* convulsion associated with these symptoms.
　　(b) **True** This is the name given to the transitional phase.
　　(c) **True** The perinatal mortality is 56/1000 births.
　　(d) **False** It is the consequence of cerebral oedema and irritation.
　　(e) **False** Delivery is the correct treatment for this condition, but stabilization with magnesium sulphate (in preference to diazepam) is usually required first.

102 (a) **False** Haemorrhage is the leading worldwide cause, and PE is the leading UK cause.
　　(b) **True**
　　(c) **False** Treatment involves cardiopulmonary resuscitation, oxygen and heparin.
　　(d) **True** This is a rare but serious differential with a high mortality.
　　(e) **False** They occur more frequently in the puerperium.

PSYCHIATRIC DISORDERS IN PREGNANCY

103 Psychiatric disease in pregnancy:

    (a) Psychosocial factors are important in the aetiology of 'baby blues'
    (b) Schizophrenics should be maintained on their usual medication
    (c) Lithium is usually stopped in pregnancy and for breastfeeding
    (d) Puerperal psychosis occurs after 3% of deliveries
    (e) The risk of recurrence of major postnatal depression is 1:10

103 (a) **True** Biological factors are important in the aetiology of severe illness.
   (b) **True** Neuroleptics are safe in pregnancy and when breastfeeding.
   (c) **True** Close monitoring of the mental state in pregnancy is required.
   (d) **False** The prevalence is about 0.2%.
   (e) **False** The recurrence risk is as high as 1:2 to 1:3.

PSYCHIATRIC DISORDERS IN PREGNANCY

NEONATOLOGY

104 Cephalhaematoma:

    (a) Is caused by oedema of the subcutaneous layers of the scalp

    (b) Should be treated by aspiration

    (c) Most commonly lies over the occipital bone

    (d) Does not vary in tension with crying

    (e) May result in ossification and asymmetry of the skull

105 Respiratory distress syndrome (RDS):

    (a) Usually occurs in infants born before week 34 of gestation

    (b) Is more common in babies born by Caesarean section

    (c) Is more common in babies born to diabetic women

    (d) Leads to cyanosis

    (e) Is treated by giving 100% oxygen

106 The following are thought to protect against hyaline membrane disease in the neonate:

    (a) Intrauterine growth retardation

    (b) Severe pre-eclampsia

    (c) Heroin addiction

    (d) Prolonged rupture of the membranes

    (e) Diabetes

104 (a) **False** It is a subperiosteal haematoma.
  (b) **False** This may lead to infection.
  (c) **False** It is usually over the parietal bones.
  (d) **True**
  (e) **True** More commonly complete absorption occurs.

105 (a) **True** After 34 weeks, the fetal lung is generally mature.
  (b) **False** As long as delivery is at term, Caesarean section does not predispose to this condition.
  (c) **True** Maternal diabetes predisposes to fetal lung immaturity.
  (d) **True** This is due to shunting of blood through unventilated areas.
  (e) **False** The oxygen concentration should be kept to the minimum necessary to relieve cyanosis.

106 (a) **True**
  (b) **True** These conditions all stress the fetus and promote surfactant production.
  (c) **True**
  (d) **True**
  (e) **False** Surfactant production is retarded in this condition.

MEDICO-LEGAL ASPECTS OF OBSTETRICS

107 To avoid potential medico-legal problems in breech delivery:

    (a) All breeches should be delivered by Caesarean section
    (b) The parents should be given the choice of mode of delivery
    (c) Ultrasound assessment of fetal size should be undertaken
    (d) X-ray pelvimetry is advisable
    (e) An epidural anaesthetic should be used

108 Home confinement is a potential source of litigation because:

    (a) There are inadequate facilities
    (b) There are unskilled attendants
    (c) Doctors are reluctant to attend such a confinement
    (d) There may be delay in obtaining skilled medical help
    (e) No mechanism exists for proper selection of cases

107 (a) **False** Litigation may just as readily rise from Caesarean section and its complications.
   (b) **False** An explanation and information should be given to the patient, but a recommendation of the mode of delivery should be given.
   (c) **True** Vaginal delivery of very large and very small breech babies is more hazardous.
   (d) **True** This is particularly so in a primigravid breech, and is usually performed at 36 weeks' gestation.
   (e) **False** The advantages of pain relief may be offset by the loss of bearing-down sensation in the second stage.

108 (a) **False** Only low-risk cases should be booked for home confinement.
   (b) **False** There is a statutory requirement to make available fully qualified midwives.
   (c) **False** General practitioners have a statutory duty to attend if called.
   (d) **True** The time factor may be crucial in dealing with an emergency at home.
   (e) **False** Doctors may advise on the suitability of a case for home confinement.

CHAPTER THREE

Gynaecology SAQs

The following short-answer questions are categorized according to the related chapters in the Ten Teachers' Texts.

DISORDERS OF THE MENSTRUAL CYCLE

1   A 42-year-old woman presents with a 6-month history of irregular menorrhagia. A urinary pregnancy test performed by her GP is negative.

(a) What investigations would you consider?   **5 marks**
(b) If the results are normal, what is the diagnosis?   **1 mark**
(c) What are the options for treatment?   **3 marks**
(d) If the scan shows uterine fibroids, what are the treatment options?   **2 marks**

FERTILITY CONTROL

2   A 36-year-old woman is requesting sterilization. She asks the following questions.

(a) What is the failure rate?   **1 mark**
(b) How do you get to my tubes?   **3 marks**
(c) How do you 'block' my tubes?   **3 marks**
(d) Are there any complications?   **3 marks**
(e) Is there anything else I should know?   **4 marks**

INFERTILITY

3   A 34-year-old woman has been unable to conceive after 2 years of trying. She has always had very irregular menstrual cycles, and a recent laparoscopy showed that her tubes were patent. Her partner's semen analysis is normal.

(a) What is she likely to be suffering from?   **1 mark**
(b) What other symptoms/signs may she have to support your diagnosis?   **3 marks**
(c) What other tests would you carry out to confirm your diagnosis?   **3 marks**
(d) Why is she unable to conceive?   **1 mark**
(e) How will you treat this couple's infertility?   **4 marks**

1 (a) Cervical smear, full blood count, coagulation screen, thyroid function tests, pelvic ultrasound scan, endometrial biopsy, hysteroscopy, and dilatation and curettage (D & C).
   (b) Dysfunctional uterine bleeding.
   (c) Cyclical progestagens, tranexamic acid, mefanamic acid, progestagen-containing IUCD.
   (d) Myomectomy, subtotal abdominal hysterectomy, total abdominal hysterectomy.

2 (a) 1 in 300.
   (b) Laparoscopy, mini-laparotomy or posterior colpotomy.
   (c) Filshie clips, Falope rings or salpingectomy.
   (d) Increased likelihood of ectopic pregnancy if the sterilization fails and the woman becomes pregnant. Increased risk of menorrhagia. Complications of anaesthesia and laparoscopy.
   (e) General anaesthesia is required. It is a day-case procedure. Vasectomy is an alternative which must be considered. If the woman wants to become pregnant in the future, it is unlikely that she will be accepted for reversal of sterilization.

3 (a) Polycystic ovarian syndrome.
   (b) Obesity, hirsutism, acne.
   (c) Pelvic ultrasound to demonstrate polycystic ovaries. LH/FSH levels (an inverted LH to FSH ratio of 2–3:1 is characteristic of this condition). Hormone profile (progesterone, testosterone, androstenedione, sex-hormone-binding globulin).
   (d) She is having anovulatory cycles.
   (e) Clomiphene or tamoxifen. Ovulation induction with ovarian down-regulation (LHRH analogues) followed by FSH treatment. In cases that are resistant to medical treatment, ovarian diathermy or laser treatment may be used.

DISORDERS OF EARLY PREGNANCY

4   A 24-year-old woman presents with vaginal bleeding and a positive home pregnancy test.

(a) What are your differential diagnoses?   **4 marks**
(b) What factors would predispose towards ectopic pregnancy?   **5 marks**
(c) What signs of ectopic pregnancy may this woman have?   **5 marks**
(d) What investigations might you perform to confirm the
    diagnosis of ectopic pregnancy?   **4 marks**
(e) What are the treatment options for ectopic pregnancy?   **3 marks**

BENIGN DISEASE OF THE UTERUS AND CERVIX

5   A sexually active 23-year-old woman's cervical smear is reported to have mild dyskaryosis.

(a) What is dyskaryosis?   **2 marks**
(b) What is the correct follow-up for this abnormality?   **3 marks**
(c) Which smear abnormalities would you refer for urgent
    colposcopy?   **3 marks**
(d) What is dysplasia?   **2 marks**
(e) How may cervical abnormalities that are detected at
    colposcopy be treated?   **4 marks**
(f) What symptoms may a woman expect after such treatment?   **1 mark**

4 (a) Threatened miscarriage, complete/incomplete miscarriage, ectopic pregnancy.

  (b) History of previous ectopic pregnancy, pelvic inflammatory disease, infertility or pelvic surgery. Current use of progesterone or IUCD contraception.

  (c) Tachycardia, hypotension, abdominal tenderness, guarding and rebound, cervical excitation, adnexal mass.

  (d) Full blood count, group and save, βhCG, pelvic ultrasound, diagnostic laparoscopy.

  (e) Surgical treatment: access through laparotomy or laparoscopy, procedure of salpingectomy or salpingostomy. Medical treatment with methotrexate. Expectant management if βhCG levels are falling, the woman is stable and the trophoblast is thought to be in regression.

5 (a) Dyskaryosis is a cellular or cytological diagnosis made from a cervical smear based on the degree of cellular atypia, and it is graded as mild, moderate or severe.

  (b) Mild dyskaryosis may revert spontaneously to normal. The smear should be repeated in 6 months' time. If the repeat smear shows persistent abnormality, the patient should be referred for colposcopy, when a biopsy diagnosis will be made and further treatment and follow-up arranged.

  (c) Moderate and severe dyskaryosis, and the presence of frankly malignant cells on cervical cytology.

  (d) Dysplasia is a tissue diagnosis made on histology of a directed biopsy obtained at colposcopy.

  (e) Large-loop excision of the transformation zone (LLETZ), laser, cold coagulation, knife cone.

  (f) She will have a bloodstained vaginal discharge that may persist for up to 2 weeks. During this time, she should avoid sexual intercourse and the use of tampons.

ENDOMETRIOSIS

6   A 32-year-old woman has a diagnosis of endometriosis made on diagnostic laparoscopy for infertility.

(a)	What is the cause of endometriosis?	3 marks
(b)	What symptoms may she have experienced?	3 marks
(c)	Can endometriosis be the cause of her infertility?	1 mark
(d)	What are the medical treatment options available?	4 marks
(e)	What are the side-effects of danazol?	5 marks

BENIGN DISEASE OF THE OVARY

7   A 24-year-old woman is admitted with severe right iliac fossa and lower abdominal pain. A pregnancy test is negative and a large right adnexal mass is easily felt on vaginal examination.

(a)	What are the possible origins of the pelvic mass?	4 marks
(b)	What are the complications of an ovarian cyst?	3 marks
(c)	What are dermoid cysts of the ovary?	2 marks
(d)	How may the diagnosis be confirmed without surgery?	1 mark
(e)	What is the appropriate management for suspected ovarian torsion?	3 marks

MALIGNANT DISEASE OF THE UTERUS AND CERVIX

8   A 56-year-old woman presents with postmenopausal bleeding.

(a)	What is the most likely cause of her symptom?	2 marks
(b)	What investigations will you perform?	3 marks
(c)	What pathology may be detected on biopsy?	3 marks
(d)	What types of endometrial hyperplasia may be diagnosed?	2 marks
(e)	What is the correct management of endometrial cancer?	2 marks
(f)	How does this cancer spread?	1 mark
(g)	What follow-up is required?	1 mark

6 (a) Retrograde menstruation is believed to be the most likely aetiology. Other presumed aetiologies include vascular spread, immune modulation and embryonic seeding.

   (b) Lower abdominal pain, dysmenorrhoea, menorrhagia and deep dyspareunia.

   (c) Endometriosis is found in about 15% of women with infertility. There is an association between infertility and endometriosis, although this does not prove that it is causal in all cases.

   (d) Danazol, continuous progestogens, continuous combined oral contraceptive pill, LHRH analogues.

   (e) Headaches, acne, hirsutism, voice changes (which may be permanent), pregnancy should be avoided.

7 (a) Ovarian cyst (corpus luteum or dermoid), uterine fibroids, pyosalpinx, hydrosalpinx, appendix abscess.

   (b) Ovarian torsion, ovarian cyst rupture, haemorrhage into an ovarian cyst.

   (c) They are the most common ovarian tumours in women of reproductive age. They are germ-cell tumours which are usually benign, commonly bilateral and typically may contain hair and teeth.

   (d) An abdominal X-ray may demonstrate the presence of teeth.

   (e) Immediate confirmation of the diagnosis by laparoscopy, and cystectomy if the ovary is still viable or oophorectomy if the ovary is necrosed. These procedures may be performed either by laparotomy or laparoscopically.

8 (a) Vulval/vaginal atrophy, although endometrial cancer must be excluded.

   (b) Pelvic ultrasound, outpatient endometrial biopsy, hysteroscopy and endometrial biopsy.

   (c) Endometrial polyp, endometrial hyperplasia, endometrial carcinoma.

   (d) Benign cystic or complex atypical endometrial hyperplasia.

   (e) Total abdominal hysterectomy and bilateral oophorectomy.

   (f) Direct spread of malignancy.

   (g) Annual vaginal vault smears.

MALIGNANT DISEASE OF THE OVARY

9   A 70-year-old woman presents with a four month history of weight-loss and a very distended abdomen.

   (a) What initial investigations would you consider?   **4 marks**
   (b) How does ovarian cancer spread?   **1 mark**
   (c) How is ovarian cancer treated?   **3 marks**
   (d) What adjuvant therapy may be used?   **2 marks**
   (e) What screening is available for ovarian cancer?   **3 marks**

CONDITIONS AFFECTING THE VULVA AND VAGINA

10   A 71-year-old woman with a vulval lesion has a biopsy which reveals lichen sclerosus.

   (a) What type of vulval disorder is lichen sclerosus?   **2 marks**
   (b) What are the common symptoms of lichen sclerosus?   **3 marks**
   (c) What are the typical signs of this condition?   **2 marks**
   (d) What are the treatment options?   **3 marks**
   (e) What is the long-term prognosis?   **2 marks**

INCONTINENCE

11   A 76-year-old woman presents with frequency of micurition, nocturia, urgency and urge incontinence.

   (a) What are the possible diagnoses?   **3 marks**
   (b) What investigations should be performed?   **3 marks**
   (c) What are the treatment options for detrusor instability?   **3 marks**
   (d) What are the treatment options for genuine stress incontinence?   **3 marks**

9 (a) Pelvic/abdominal ultrasound, full blood count, urea and electrolytes, liver function tests, CA125, intravenous urogram, CT scan.
   (b) Transperitoneal/ascitic spread.
   (c) Total abdominal hysterectomy, bilateral salpingo-oophorectomy and omentectomy. The principle of surgical treatment is to debulk the tumour as much as possible. Surgery involves a vertical incision.
   (d) The most effective chemotherapy involves platinum compounds. These are used either as single agents or in combination with other agents.
   (e) Screening programmes involving family history, tumour markers and pelvic ultrasound are being explored at present. None of these modalities has yet been established as effective.

10 (a) Lichen sclerosus is a non-neoplastic epithelial vulval disorder (these include lichen sclerosus, squamous-cell hyperplasia and other dermatoses).
   (b) Burning/itching of the vulva, white areas on the vulva (leukoplakia) and superficial dyspareunia.
   (c) White vulval plaques and vulval atrophy.
   (d) Topical corticosteroids, oestrogen or testosterone cream. Surgery is not useful in this condition.
   (e) The disease may be refractory to treatment and may progress to malignancy in about 5% of cases.

11 (a) Urinary tract infection, detrusor instability, genuine stress incontinence.
   (b) Urine microscopy, culture and sensitivity (MCS), random blood sugar, urodynamics.
   (c) Bladder drill, anticholinergics, calcium-channel blockers, tricyclic antidepressants.
   (d) Pelvic floor exercises, maximal electrical therapy, faradism, bladder neck suspension surgery.

PROLAPSE

12   A 62-year-old woman presents with a uterine prolapse.

   (a) How is uterine prolapse classified?   **3 marks**
   (b) What symptoms may the patient have?   **5 marks**
   (c) What other problems may be associated with uterine
      prolapse?   **4 marks**
   (d) What treatment options may the patient be offered?   **2 marks**

MENOPAUSE

13   A 52-year-old woman has climacteric symptoms.

   (a) What types of symptoms may she have?   **6 marks**
   (b) What diseases may HRT prevent?   **3 marks**
   (c) How may HRT be given?   **4 marks**
   (d) What are the contraindications to HRT?   **4 marks**
   (e) How long should HRT be prescribed for?   **1 mark**

PROLAPSE

12 (a) First degree: uterine descent confined within the vagina. Second degree: uterine descent with cervix outside the introitus but the body still within the vagina. Third degree: uterine body descends to outside the introitus.

   (b) Vaginal lump, backache, dragging sensation in the vagina, urinary frequency and nocturia, incontinence, digitation, bloody vaginal discharge.

   (c) Cystocele, enterocele, rectocele, urethrocele.

   (d) Vaginal pessary, vaginal hysterectomy.

13 (a) Psychological and vasomotor effects: hot flushes, night sweats, irritability, poor memory, lack of concentration, decreased libido, and depression. Local genital effects: genital tract atrophy and dyspareunia.

   (b) Osteoporosis, cardiovascular disease, Alzheimer's disease.

   (c) Tablets, transdermal patches, hormone gel, implants.

   (d) Breast cancer, coexisting deep venous thrombosis or pulmonary embolus, active liver disease, post-menopausal bleeding.

   (e) HRT needs to be used for a minimum of 10 years to have significant long-term benefits.

CHAPTER FOUR

Obstetric SAQs

The following short-answer questions are categorized according to the related chapters in the Ten Teachers' Texts.

ULTRASOUND IMAGING AND FETAL ASSESSMENT

1   A woman known to have a small-for-gestational-age (SGA) fetus is admitted to hospital for further monitoring.

  (a) What are the causes of SGA fetuses?   **4 marks**
  (b) What is a biophysical profile?   **5 marks**
  (c) What would constitute an abnormal umbilical artery Doppler result?   **3 marks**
  (d) What are the neonatal complications of a growth-restricted baby?   **4 marks**
  (e) What are the long-term complications of intrauterine growth restriction?   **4 marks**

ANTENATAL CARE

2   A 28-year-old West-Indian woman books for shared antenatal care in her first pregnancy.

  (a) What screening is performed on the booking bloods?   **6 marks**
  (b) What is the purpose of routine ultrasound scans?   **4 marks**
  (c) How is screening for gestational diabetes performed?   **3 marks**
  (d) What is the purpose of the physical examination at each of the antenatal visits?   **2 marks**

LABOUR

3   A primigravid woman is admitted in labour at term. Despite contracting strongly and frequently with intact membranes, she only progresses from 4 to 5 cm over the next 4 hours.

  (a) What is the diagnosis?   **1 mark**
  (b) What are the common causes of this condition?   **3 marks**
  (c) What may be done to accelerate the progress of labour?   **1 mark**
  (d) Two hours later, the cervix is unchanged. What should be done next?   **1 mark**
  (e) If labour had progressed normally until 7 cm, where progress stopped, what would be the diagnosis?   **1 mark**
  (f) What are the causes of this condition?   **3 marks**

1 (a) Incorrect dating, constitutionally small fetus, abnormally small fetus (uteroplacental insufficiency and fetal abnormality).
   (b) Ultrasound scan for liquor volume, fetal tone, fetal movements and breathing movements. A CTG or Doppler is also usually performed.
   (c) Placental insufficiency increases the placental vascular resistance, and Doppler of the umbilical artery shows an increased resistance index. When severe, end diastolic flow may be absent or reversed.
   (d) Hypoglycaemia, hypothermia, poor feeding, necrotizing enterocolitis, pulmonary hypoplasia (if delivered prematurely).
   (e) Adult hypertensive and cardiovascular disease, diabetes mellitus, chronic lung disease.

2 (a) Haemoglobin concentration, haemoglobinopathy screen, blood group, syphilis screen, rubella and hepatitis status.
   (b) Dating the pregnancy, placental localization, fetal growth and fetal abnormality (cardiac, neural tube and chromosomal).
   (c) Urine testing, random or postprandial blood sugar and modified glucose tolerance testing.
   (d) Blood pressure to check for pre-eclampsia, abdominal palpation to check fetal growth and presentation.

3 (a) Primary dysfunctional labour.
   (b) Inco-ordinate uterine activity, malposition (i.e. occipito-posterior position), malpresentation.
   (c) Rupture of the amniotic membranes.
   (d) A syntocinon infusion should be started.
   (e) Secondary arrest.
   (f) Malposition, malpresentation or cephalopelvic disproportion.

THE PUERPERIUM

4   A woman becomes pyrexial (38.7°C) 5 days after an emergency
    Caesarean section.

(a) What are the possible causes of her pyrexia?	**6 marks**
(b) What symptoms may she have?	**5 marks**
(c) What clinical signs may be present?	**5 marks**
(d) What investigations might you perform?	**4 marks**

PRE-ECLAMPSIA AND GROWTH RESTRICTION

5   A primigravid woman is admitted at 28 weeks' gestation with a
    blood pressure of 160/105 mmHg and ++ proteinuria. Her pre-
    pregnancy blood pressure was 110/60 mmHg.

(a) What is the likely diagnosis?	**1 mark**
(b) What symptoms may she have?	**5 marks**
(c) What investigations would you want to perform?	**6 marks**
(d) What haematological complications may the patient develop?	**3 marks**
(e) What is the cure for this condition?	**2 marks**

PRENATAL DIAGNOSIS

6   Chromosomal abnormal pregnancies.

(a) What screening tests are available for Down's syndrome?	**4 marks**
(b) What diagnostic tests are available for this condition and when are they performed?	**6 marks**
(c) What are the complications of invasive prenatal testing?	**4 marks**
(d) Name some common aneuploidies.	**5 marks**

THE PUERPERIUM

4 (a) Infection of the breast, chest, wound, endometrium or urinary tract, or deep venous thrombosis.
   (b) Breast engorgement and pain, abdominal pain, pain in the Caesarean scar, discharging wound, offensive lochia, urinary frequency and dysuria, calf pain/swelling, chest pain and cough.
   (c) Engorged and tender breasts, red, indurated and discharging wound, swollen, tender calves, tender uterus.
   (d) Urine for MCS, wound swab, high vaginal swab, blood culture, Doppler of the calf, chest X-ray and ECG.

5 (a) Pre-eclampsia or proteinuric pregnancy-induced hypertension.
   (b) Headaches, visual disturbances, abdominal pain, nausea and vomiting, confusion and irritability.
   (c) Blood tests: full blood count, urea and electrolytes, liver function tests, coagulation profile. Urine: 24 hour collection for protein estimation. Fetal: ultrasound for growth, biophysical profile and Doppler.
   (d) Thrombocytopenia, haemolysis, disseminated intravascular coagulation.
   (e) The cure is delivery, but in this case antihypertensives may be used to prolong the pregnancy for long enough to allow improved neonatal survival.

6 (a) Maternal age, biochemical screening, nuchal translucency, anomaly scanning.
   (b) Chorionic villus sampling (CVS) (>11 weeks), amniocentesis (>15 weeks) and cordocentesis (>20 weeks).
   (c) Miscarriage, culture failure, limb reduction defects if CVS is performed too early, talipes and respiratory problems if amniocentesis is performed too early.
   (d) Down's (trisomy 21), Edward's (trisomy 18), Patau's (trisomy 13), Turner's (45XO) and Klienfelter's syndrome (47XXY).

MULTIPLE PREGNANCY

7   A woman has a first-trimester scan which shows a twin pregnancy.

    (a) What is the difference between zygosity and chorionicity?   **2 marks**
    (b) Which types of twins are associated with an increased risk of complications ?   **1 mark**
    (c) How can chorionicity be diagnosed on ultrasound?   **2 marks**
    (d) What complications are more likely to occur in monochorionic twins?   **4 marks**
    (e) How may twin-to-twin transfusion be identified antenatally?   **4 marks**
    (f) What options are available for managing twin-to-twin transfusion?   **2 marks**

ANTENATAL OBSTETRIC COMPLICATIONS

8   A 25-year-old woman is admitted at 35 weeks' gestation with severe abdominal pain and vaginal bleeding. On examination, her pulse is 110 beats/minute, blood pressure is 110/50 mmHg and her uterus is tender and irritable.

    (a) What is the diagnosis?   **1 mark**
    (b) Why is this not bleeding from a placenta praevia?   **1 mark**
    (c) What is the immediate management of this condition?   **6 marks**
    (d) When should the fetus be delivered?   **2 marks**
    (e) How should the fetus be delivered?   **1 mark**

PERINATAL INFECTIONS

9   A 26-year-old woman is found to have beta-haemolytic *Streptococcus* on a high vaginal swab performed at 28 weeks for vaginal irritation.

    (a) What is the prevalence of group B *Streptococcus* carriage?   **1 mark**
    (b) Should this be treated now?   **2 marks**
    (c) What is the fetal/neonatal risk?   **1 mark**
    (d) What should be done if this patient has prelabour rupture of the membranes?   **2 marks**
    (e) When should she be treated?   **2 marks**

7 (a) Monozygotic twins originate from one oocyte (identical).
       Monozygotic twins may go on to be monochorionic (share one
       placenta) or dichorionic (have two placentae).
   (b) Monochorionic twins have a higher spontaneous miscarriage and
       perinatal mortality rate.
   (c) The lambda sign is characteristic of dichorionic fused placentae, and
       the T-sign is seen in monochorionic twins.
   (d) Congenital malformations, intrauterine growth retardation, preterm
       delivery, twin-to-twin transfusion.
   (e) Clinical signs: polydypsia, acute hydramnios. Ultrasound features:
       donor twin is growth retarded with anhydramnios, and recipient
       twin is larger, with hydrops and polyhydramnios.
   (f) Amniodrainage or fetoscopic laser ablation of the inter-connecting
       placental vessels.

8 (a) Placental abruption.
   (b) Placenta praevia causes painless bleeding.
   (c) IV access, full blood count, blood crossmatch, coagulation profile,
       regular pulse/blood pressure monitoring, fetal monitoring; alert
       anaesthetists and haematologists.
   (d) An abruption large enough to cause tachycardia and hypotension
       warrants immediate delivery.
   (e) Vaginal delivery if the mother and fetus are uncompromised, but in
       this situation a Caesarean section should be performed.

9 (a) Around 15–20% of women are asymptomatic carriers.
   (b) No, as this is a commensal and not a pathogen in the vagina. The
       vagina will also be recolonized soon after treatment is stopped.
   (c) Approximately,1 in every 1000 neonates will suffer serious neonatal
       complications from group B *Streptococcus* septicaemia.
   (d) If a high vaginal swab is positive, antibiotic treatment and delivery
       should be advocated.
   (e) The mother will require intravenous antibiotics in labour, and the
       baby should be given prophylactic antibiotics.

MEDICAL DISEASES COMPLICATING PREGNANCY

10   A known diabetic on insulin attends your surgery.

(a) What should she do in the pre-pregnancy period?   **1 mark**
(b) What are the main effects of pregnancy on the diabetes?   **1 mark**
(c) What are the main effects of the diabetes on the fetus?   **4 marks**
(d) How is this condition managed in labour?   **4 marks**

PRETERM LABOUR

11   A 22-year-old woman presents at 26 weeks' gestation with a history of leaking fluid per vaginum.

(a) How is rupture of membranes diagnosed?   **3 marks**
(b) What are the complications of rupture of membranes?   **3 marks**
(c) How should the pregnancy be monitored?   **6 marks**
(d) How can the outcome be improved?   **2 marks**

OBSTETRIC EMERGENCIES

12   A woman is bleeding actively soon after delivery of the placenta.

(a) What is the immediate management?   **3 marks**
(b) How would you attempt to arrest the bleeding?   **4 marks**
(c) What is the diagnosis if more than 500 mL of blood are lost?   **1 mark**
(d) What are the causes of this condition?   **4 marks**
(e) If bleeding does not arrest, what may have occurred?   **1 mark**

PSYCHIATRIC DISORDERS IN PREGNANCY

13   A 25-year-old mother is weepy and miserable.

(a) What is the most likely diagnosis?   **1 mark**
(b) What other symptoms might she have?   **4 marks**
(c) What is the appropriate investigation for this condition?   **1 mark**
(d) How is this condition treated?   **2 marks**
(e) What are the other two less common psychiatric
     complications of the puerperium?   **2 marks**

10 (a) Tight diabetic control during the periconceptual period reduces the fetal risks.
   (b) Pregnancy hormones are gluconeogenic, resulting in increased insulin requirements in pregnancy.
   (c) Congenital abnormality (especially cardiac), fetal macrosomia, polyhydramnios, late stillbirth.
   (d) Insulin sliding scale and glucose IV infusion in labour, and resumption of pre-pregnancy insulin doses when the mother resumes her normal diet post-delivery. Close neonatal observations for hypoglycaemia.

11 (a) Speculum examination, nitrazine or fibronectin test.
   (b) Preterm labour, intrauterine infection, respiratory distress syndrome.
   (c) Four-hourly maternal temperature and pulse, daily abdominal palpation and inspection of the vaginal discharge, weekly white cell counts and C-reactive protein and daily CTG.
   (d) Prolonging the pregnancy as long as possible, and antenatal steroid administration.

12 (a) Intravenous access, group and crossmatch, intravenous fluid.
   (b) Rub the uterus to stimulate contractions, use syntocinon, ergometrine or carboprost to help uterine contractions, check that the placenta is complete. Empty the bladder.
   (c) Primary postpartum haemorrhage.
   (d) Uterine atony, retained placental tissue, trauma to the lower genital tract, ruptured uterus.
   (e) Disseminated vascular coagulation may have developed.

13 (a) Postpartum or baby blues.
   (b) Anxiety, labile mood, insomnia, poor appetite.
   (c) This is a diagnosis made on the basis of the maternal history.
   (d) Support and reassurance are the mainstay of management.
   (e) Postpartum depression and psychosis.

CHAPTER FIVE

Core Tutorials

The following 10 core problems are intended to cover the key topics in under-graduate obstetrics and gynaecology. Each core problem involves a clinical scenario linked to four or five key topics. These core problems are ideal for group study, learning and assessment. Students are advised to revise the key topics before discussing the answers to the clinical questions posed.

CORE PROBLEM 1: OBSTETRIC TRAGEDIES

A woman is in premature labour at 26 weeks. She had a previous neonatal death after delivery at the same gestation.

Key topics

- Assessment of gestational age
- Antenatal care
- Obstetric statistics
- Tests of fetal well-being
- Premature labour

Assessment of gestational age

1 Is assessment of gestational age important?
Neonatal mortality and morbidity are determined mainly by gestational age. For example, survival at 26 weeks is approximately 70%, and it rises by 2% for every day beyond this gestation. All obstetric interventions are dependent on gestation, including visits, blood tests, investigations and operations.

2 Discuss dating of pregnancy by ultrasound scan (USS) vs. last menstrual period (LMP).
LMP is often inaccurate because of forgotten or incorrect dates. In addition, irregular cycles and conception while on or recently having stopped the pill or while breastfeeding will affect the estimation of gestation. When the LMP is known with a regular 28-day cycle, estimated date of delivery (EDD) = LMP + 1 year 7 days − 3 months (Nägele's rule). USS is more accurate than LMP dates.

3 When is USS assessment of gestational age best performed?
First-trimester scans are better than second-trimester scans (rate of growth is highest). Estimated date of delivery by early pregnancy scan (crown–rump length) is accurate to within ± 5 days; 20-week scan (biparietal diameter) is accurate to within ± 12 days.

Antenatal care

1 What type of antenatal care would you recommend for this patient?
Full hospital care lead by obstetrician with regular visits every 2–4 weeks would be better than shared or community care.

2 Discuss the different types of antenatal care.
Community care/shared care/full hospital care. Risk assessment at initial booking visit with providers of antenatal care (midwife, GP, obstetrician).
● Community care – GP, midwife;
● Shared care – GP, obstetrician, midwife;
● Full hospital care – obstetrician, midwife.
Traditional shared care visits: 4 weekly until 28 weeks; fortnightly until 36 weeks; once weekly thereafter.

Obstetric statistics

1 Define term pregnancy.
A term pregnancy occurs between 37 and 42 completed weeks' gestation.

2 What proportion of women deliver before 37 weeks?
Preterm delivery occurs in 6–10% of pregnancies, but accounts for up to 75% of all perinatal deaths.

3 Discuss the problems of extreme prematurity for the neonate.
● Mortality depends on gestation.
● Morbidity: respiratory distress syndrome (RDS), chronic lung disease, hypothermia, feeding problems, infection, intraventricular haemorrhage (IVH), necrotizing enterocolitis (NEC), jaundice, retinopathy of the newborn, hearing problems.

4 How do survival rates vary with gestation?
The fetus is considered to be viable at 24 weeks, with a mortality rate of 50%. Survival rates increase by 2% each day thereafter to 80% between 26 and 27 weeks, reaching 90% at between 28 and 29 weeks.

5 What is the role of antenatal steroids?
They induce surfactant production and improve fetal lung maturity, thereby reducing the incidence of respiratory distress syndrome (the commonest and most significant problem of prematurity).

Tests of fetal well-being

1 Compare the assessment of fetal size by palpation vs. ultrasound.
Symphysis–fundal height (SFH) measurement detects only 50% of small fetuses, but SFH remains the only objective clinical method. Between 26 and

36 weeks, SFH (in cm) = number of weeks' gestation ± 2 cm. Ultrasound is more accurate (to within ±15% in fetal size estimation).

2   Describe the differences between 'reactive' and 'unreactive' CTG.
Normal (reactive) cardiotocograph (CTG) parameters: baseline, 110–150 beats/min; short-term baseline variability 5–10 beats/min, with accelerations (>2 in 20 mins) and no decelerations. Unreactive CTG: abnormal baseline rate, reduced baseline variability, no accelerations or the presence of decelerations.

3   How do we assess fetal well-being on ultrasound (USS)?
USS assesses fetal size/velocity (one USS looks at fetal size, and two scans at least 2 weeks apart look at growth velocity) and biophysical profile (BPP). BPP is the combination of fetal movements and tone, liquor volume, breathing movements and Doppler assessment of placental and fetal blood flow.

Premature labour

1   Define labour and premature labour.
Labour is defined as the onset of regular painful contractions associated with cervical dilatation and descent of the presenting part. Rupture of membranes or a 'show' are not required to diagnose labour.
  Premature labour is defined as labour occurring before 37 weeks.

2   What are the risk factors for premature delivery?
Major risk factors: previous premature delivery, multiple pregnancy, polyhydramnios, cervical incompetence, abnormally shaped uterus, abdominal surgery in pregnancy, iatrogenic factors (pre-eclampsia or intrauterine growth restriction, for example).
Minor risk factors: irritable uterus (e.g. from bleeding), preterm spontaneous rupture of membranes, infection, fibroids, maternal sepsis, pre-existing maternal disease (e.g. diabetes, renal disease, antiphospholipid syndrome).

3   What is the role of tocolytics in the management of premature labour?
To delay the delivery by 24–48 hours to give antenatal steroids time to work, and to allow transfer of the mother to a unit with neonatal facilities. Side-effects of tocolysis include tremor, palpitations, dizziness, tachycardia, hypotension, hyperglycaemia, hypokalaemia and cardiac failure.

CORE PROBLEM 2: PRENATAL SCREENING

A 34-year-old woman with a twin pregnancy requests screening for Down's syndrome.

Key topics

- Chromosome abnormalities
- Single-gene defects
- Anatomical defects
- Twin pregnancy
- Obstetric operations

Chromosomal abnormalities vs. single-gene defects

1 Discuss the differences between chromosomal abnormalities and single-gene defects.

Chromosomal abnormalities involve an altered number of chromosomes (also known as aneuploidy) or a deletion/translocation/inversion of the chromosome. These are detected by chromosomal analysis.

Single-gene defects have the normal number and structure of chromosomes, but usually contain a small mutation in a single gene, resulting in an abnormal protein chain product. These require DNA analysis for detection.

2 Give some common examples of these defects.

Single-gene defects: often autosomal recessive disorders such as cystic fibrosis, thalassaemia, sickle-cell disorder and Tay-Sachs' disease.

Chromsomal defects. Trisomies: 21 = Down's, 18 = Edward's, 13 = Patau's. Monosomies: 45XO = Turner's. Triploidy: 67XXX = incompatible with life.

3 What is the difference between screening and diagnosis?

Screening assesses the risk, whereas diagnosis confirms the presence of abnormality.

4 What are the currently available screening tests for Down's syndrome?

Maternal age, triple or serum screening test, nuchal translucency scan and the anomaly scan at 20 weeks.

5 Discuss the timing and possible complications of diagnostic tests.

Chorion villus sampling: from 11–40 weeks; results are obtained in a few days – hence the option of early surgical termination of pregnancy, but higher laboratory failure rate (mosaicism).

Amniocentesis: from 15–40 weeks; full results are not available for 3 weeks, hence late medical termination of pregnancy (mini-labour).

Both invasive methods have a 1% procedure-related risk of miscarriage.

Anatomical defects

1   What are the commonest major congenital abnormalities?
Neural-tube defects and cardiac abnormality.

2   Discuss the value of a routine anomaly scan.
It assesses normal fetal anatomy and size, detects most major structural defects, confirms the estimated date of delivery and localizes the placental site.

3   What is the value of prenatal detection of congenital defects?
Detection of potential chromosomal or structural problems associated with poor fetal outcome gives the parents the option of terminating the pregnancy.

Detection of structural problems which will require corrective surgery postnatally allows appropriate counselling for the parents and planning of the pregnancy care and delivery in an appropriate unit.

Twin pregnancy

1   How is screening and diagnosis modified in twin pregnancy?
Nuchal translucency screening is unaffected in twins, whereas the triple/serum screening test is not valuable. Diagnostic tests are more difficult (double amnio/CVS with a higher risk of miscarriage). The parents are faced with a dilemma if only one twin is abnormal, as they must decide whether to terminate the whole pregnancy, have selective fetocide or continue regardless.

2   Discuss the importance of determining chorionicity in twins.
Monochorionic twins are always identical (monzygous), whereas dichorionic twins may be monozygous or dizygous. Monochorionic pregnancies have a higher risk of miscarriage, premature delivery, perinatal mortality, intrauterine growth restriction and twin–twin transfusion syndrome.

3   How is antenatal care different in twin pregnancy?
Full hospital care is required. The risk of all maternal and fetal complications (except post-term delivery) is higher.

4   Discuss the timing and management of delivery in twins.
About 75% of twins deliver by 38 weeks and 20% of twins deliver by 32 weeks' gestation.

Most twin pregnancies are induced at 38–40 weeks if they are not delivered.

The mode of delivery depends on presentation: 42% are cephalic–cephalic, 38% are cephalic–breech and 20% are breech–breech.

Management of the first stage of labour if twin 1 is cephalic is the same as for a singleton (except that there should be a continuous CTG of both twins). During management of the second stage of labour, be aware of malpresentation of twin 2 and uterine inertia resulting in a prolonged inter-twin delivery period. Active management of the third stage is necessary to prevent post-partum haemorrhage.

Obstetric operations

1   What is legally required before a termination can be performed?
The 1967 Abortion Act requires two doctors' signatures (blue form). Termination is legal up to 24 weeks' gestation, but can be performed after 24 weeks for congenital abnormality that is incompatible with life or likely to result in 'significant' handicap. The informed written consent of the mother is required. The procedure can only be performed in licensed centres. After the procedure, HSA4 (yellow form) has to be filled in by the doctor performing the procedure, legally notifying the Department of Health of the termination.

2   How can termination of pregnancy be performed?
The surgical method can be used up to 13 weeks maximum (suction evacuation under general anaesthetic). It requires cervical preparation with prostaglandins.
The medical method is usually used after 14 weeks, employing prostaglandins with or without oxytocics and antiprogesterones.

3   What are the complications of termination of pregnancy?
Bleeding, perforation of the uterus, retained products, infection, infertility, psychological effects and possible cervical incompetence.

CORE PROBLEM 3: PREGNANCY COMPLICATIONS

A 30-year-old primigravida has proteinuria and hypertension, and has had a small vaginal bleed. When should she be delivered?

Key topics

● Antenatal care
● Tests of fetal well-being
● Pregnancy hypertension
● Antepartum haemorrhage
● Obstetric operations

Antenatal care

1   How do we assess pregnancy risk at the booking visit?
Previous obstetric history: previous pregnancy complications, mode of delivery, outcome, previous gynaecological surgery, infertility treatment, etc.
Past medical history: medical disorder (e.g. diabetes, hypertension, renal problems, antiphospholipid syndrome).
Family history: hypertension, diabetes, congenital abnormalities.
Examination: blood pressure, urinanalysis, cardiovascular/respiratory system.

2   What would you check at each antenatal visit and why?
Maternal well-being: symptoms, blood pressure, urinanalysis (protein/glycosuria), general examination (anaemia, oedema, tenderness).
Fetal well-being: assessment of size (SFH), fetal movements and fetal heart rate.

3   Where would blood pressure monitoring be performed – in hospital or at home?
In this case, hospital admission would be necessary in view of the bleeding, and hypertension associated with proteinuria. In cases of mild hypertension with no other symptoms, the patient can be monitored at home.

Tests of fetal well-being

1   What is the fetal biophysical profile?
It involves the measurement of fetal movement, liquor volume, fetal tone, breathing movements and heart rate.

2   What are the possible reasons for a baby being 'small'?
Wrong dates, constitutionally small, utero-placental insufficiency or fetal abnormality (e.g. infection, chromosomal abnormality, genetic syndrome).
3   How do we assess fetal hypoxaemia in growth-restricted fetuses?
Reduced fetal movement, poor biophysical profile, unreactive CTG or abnormal/fetal Dopplers.

Pregnancy hypertension

1   What is the classification of hypertension of pregnancy?
Raised blood pressure > 140/90 on at least two occasions 4 hours apart in a previously normotensive woman or blood pressure > 160/110 mmHg with or without proteinuria occurring after 20 weeks' gestation. Raised blood pressure before 20 weeks is usually due to essential hypertension.

2   What are the maternal and fetal complications of pre-eclampsia?
Maternal complications: eclampsia, HELLP syndrome, renal failure, disseminated intravascular coagulation, abruption, adult respiratory distress syndrome, intracranial bleeding, maternal death.
Fetal complications: prematurity, intrauterine growth restriction, abruption, death (the perinatal mortality rate is 12% in eclampsia).

3   How do we assess the severity of pre-eclampsia?
Gestation at onset, blood pressure, associated degree of proteinuria, associated symptoms and signs, abnormalities of liver and renal function.

4   What is the cure for pre-eclampsia?
Delivery.

5   When would antihypertensives be used in pre-eclampsia?
At very early gestations to prolong the pregnancy and decrease the risk of prematurity for the fetus, but only if the fetus and the mother are not compromised by prolonging the pregnancy.

Antepartum haemorrhage

1   Describe the signs and symptoms of abruption vs. placenta praevia.
Placental abruption: *Pain*, uterine contractions and uterine tenderness, with or without fetal hypoxaemia or intrauterine death, uterine bleeding (concealed or revealed).
Placenta praevia: *Painless* uterine bleeding from low-lying placental bed.

2   What are the fetal and maternal risks of abruption?
Fetal risks: intrauterine growth restriction, fetal hypoxaemia, death.
Maternal risks: maternal collapse from massive blood loss, disseminated intravascular coagulation, postpartum haemorrhage, renal failure and death.

Obstetric operations

1   When would the delivery be indicated?
At term, unless by prolonging the pregnancy either the mother or the baby would be further compromised.

2   How would delivery be effected?
Ideally by vaginal delivery, unless either the mother or the baby would be further compromised by labour and delivery.

3   How is induction of labour performed?

Vaginal prostaglandins are used to ripen the cervix. If possible, artificial rupture of the membranes is performed before commencing an oxytocic infusion.

4   Would anaesthesia in women with pre-eclampsia be altered?

Epidural: ideal for reducing hypertension. Maternal thrombocytopenia (< 100) is a contraindication to epidural anaesthesia.

General anaesthesia has increased risks: difficult intubation/laryngeal oedema, aspiration, increased blood pressure response to laryngoscopy.

5   What is the difference between classical and lower segment Caesarean section?

Lower segment Caesarean section involves a transverse lower segment cut in the uterus, less bleeding, less scarring and a lower risk of rupture in a subsequent pregnancy.

Classical Caesarean section involves a vertical cut to the body of the uterus, more bleeding and scarring and a higher risk of scar rupture in a subsequent pregnancy. It is only performed in very early pregnancy when the lower segment has not formed.

CORE PROBLEM 4: BLEEDING IN EARLY PREGNANCY

A 32-year-old woman with rheumatoid arthritis has had two previous miscarriages. After missing a period for 6 weeks she has had irregular bleeding and pain for the past 3 weeks.

Key topics

- Diagnosis of pregnancy
- Miscarriage
- Trophoblastic disease

Diagnosis of pregnancy

1   What are the signs and symptoms of pregnancy?

Symptoms: amenorrhoea, breast tenderness, tiredness, urinary frequency, early morning sickness.

Signs: skin changes (palmar erythema, spider naevi, chloasma gravidarum, striae gravidarum), purple discoloration of the vagina, enlarged soft uterus, fetal movements, FH.

2 When would serum βhCG be preferred to urinary βhCG?
In cases of suspected ectopic pregnancy (when urinary βhCG can be very low, or for serial hCG measurements), suspected molar pregnancy and for follow-up after conservative/surgical/medical treatment for ectopic pregnancy to ensure complete inactivity of the trophoblast.

3 What is the role of ultrasound in the diagnosis of pregnancy?
Confirmation of intrauterine pregnancy, viability, dating, and chorionicity in twin pregnancy.

Miscarriage

1 What are the maternal risks of miscarriage or ectopic pregnancy?
Maternal mortality and morbidity: death, bleeding, sepsis, operative complications, infertility, rhesus isoimmunization, psychological trauma.

2 What are the different types of miscarriages?
Threatened: bleeding only. Inevitable: bleeding with open cervix and large uterus.
Incomplete: bleeding with open cervix and partially empty uterus.
Complete: closed cervix and small uterus. Septic abortion: any of the above, if infected. Missed abortion (blighted ovum): dead baby or empty sac on ultrasound scan.

3 Explain conservative vs. surgical management of miscarriage.
Surgery (evacuation of retained products of conception): general anaesthetic, cervical dilatation and curettage (risk of bleeding, retained products of conception, perforation, infection, Asherman's syndrome).
Conservative: await spontaneous complete miscarriage (as above, but no risk of general anaesthetic, perforation or Asherman's syndrome).

4 Why and when is anti-D used?
To prevent rhesus isoimmunization and haemolytic disease of the newborn in future pregnancies. Use anti-D with threatened miscarriage, termination of pregnancy, evacuation of retained products of conception, ectopic pregnancy, CVS/amnio, antepartum haemorrhage, external cephalic version and delivery.

5 How often and why do spontaneous miscarriages occur?
Miscarriage is pregnancy loss at < 24 weeks' gestation. It occurs in about 15% of recognized pregnancies. It is probably much more frequent, with a peak incidence at 7–8 weeks' gestation. Causes include conceptual problems (chromosomal/structural problems/abnormal placentation), maternal factors (systemic disease, infection, uterine abnormalities, immunological problems), drugs and hypersecretion of LH.

6   What is the definition of recurrent miscarriage?
Three or more consecutive first-trimester miscarriages.

7   What are the causes of recurrent miscarriage?
About 75% are unexplained. Hypersecretion of LH and antiphospholipid syndrome are the most common identifiable causes. Other causes include genetic factors, uterine abnormalities, infection, endocrine causes (insulin-dependent diabetes mellitus), and thrombophilic defects.

Trophoblastic disease

1   How does trophoblastic disease usually present?
Symptoms: irregular heavy bleeding, anaemia, hyperemesis, haemoptysis.
Signs: large uterus, grape-like tissue per vaginum, pre-eclampsia, thyro-
toxicosis, high hCG, snow-storm appearance on USS.

2   Discuss the management of molar pregnancy.
Investigations: βhCG levels, full blood count, group and save, thyroid function tests, ultrasound scan, chest X-ray.
Diagnosis: confirmed by histology (D & C).
Treatment: suction evacuation of the uterus.
Follow-up: central registration and serial HCG measurement. If there is a persistent high HCG, it will require chemotherapy (methotrexate). Follow-up is also required after future pregnancies.

3   What is choriocarcinoma?
It is a malignant tumour of the trophoblast, which may follow normal or molar pregnancy. The incidence 1 in 50 000 live births.

CORE PROBLEM 5: LABOUR COMPLICATIONS

A 25-year-old woman has been in spontaneous labour for 15 hours during week 40 of her first pregnancy. The fetal heart tracing shows occasional prolonged dips with a uterine contraction.

Key topics
- Normal labour
- Abnormal labour
- Labour monitoring
- Obstetric operations

Normal labour

1 Discuss the mechanisms of labour.

These involve the *powers* (uterine contractions, abdominal muscles, diaphragm), *passage* (bony pelvis, pelvic floor) and *passenger* (baby – size and position).

Mechanism in vertex presentation: flexion, internal rotation, descent, crowning, extension, restitution, external rotation, delivery of the body.

2 What are the stages of normal labour?

First stage: onset of labour to full dilatation of the cervix.

Second stage: full dilatation to complete expulsion of the baby.

Third stage: from delivery of the baby to delivery of the placenta.

3 Discuss the options for pain relief for this woman in labour.

Non-pharmacological options: relaxation and massage, transcutaneous electrical nerve stimulation, warm water bath.

Pharmacological options: nitrous oxide (Entonox); pethidine and other opiates; epidural.

Abnormal labour

1 What are the patterns of abnormal labour progress?

Prolonged latent phase: symptoms of labour but not yet 3 cm dilated.

Primary dysfunctional labour: more than 3 cm dilated, but progress is less than 1 cm/hour (labour never reaches the active phase).

Secondary arrest: labour reaches active phase, but then stops.

2 What are the causes of abnormal labour progress?

Primary dysfunction: abnormal uterine action (primiparae), malposition.

Secondary arrest: malposition (occipito-posterior or occipito-transverse), malpresentation (breech).

Cephalo-pelvic disproportion (CPD): true CPD is very rare. Relative CPD is a common diagnosis as a consequence of malposition or inadequate uterine activity.

3 What are the maternal and fetal risks of prolonged labour?

Maternal risks: infection, postpartum haemorrhage, thromboembolism, vesico-vaginal fistulas, psychological trauma.

Fetal risks: fetal hypoxia, meconium aspiration, infection, death.

4 Discuss the management of dystocia in labour.

Inco-ordinate uterine activity and malposition are managed with oxytocin infusion (with caution in multiparae). Malpresentations (breech) are managed expectantly or by lower-segment Caesarean section (LSCS). True cephalo-pelvic disproportion (CPD) or unresolving relative CPD is managed by LSCS.

5   What is shoulder dystocia and how is it managed?
It is an obstetric emergency. The head is delivered, but there is failure of delivery of the shoulders.

There is a risk of birth asphyxia and trauma (cerebral palsy, brachial plexus injury, fracture of the clavicle). Management (HELPER): call for senior **Help**, **E**pisiotomy, legs to **L**ithotomy, suprapubic **P**ressure, **E**nter vagina to achieve **R**otation of the shoulders manually by abduction or delivery of the posterior shoulder first.

Also call for the paediatrician and anaesthetist.

Labour monitoring

1   How is progress in labour monitored?
By means of a partogram (pictorial representation of labour progress as well as fetal/maternal well-being).

2   What is the significance of meconium?
It indicates the passage of fetal faecal matter *in utero*. It can reflect fetal hypoaxemia.

3   What is the correct management of an unreactive CTG?
Fetal blood sampling to check for the presence of fetal hypoxia (as CTGs have a high false-positive rate). Assess cervical dilatation, presence of other factors (e.g. meconium), antepartum haemorrhage and administered drugs (pethidine).

Obstetric operations

1   What are the indications for operative delivery?
Instrumental delivery
Maternal indications: maternal exhaustion, distress, conditions requiring decreased maternal effort (e.g. cardiac conditions, retinal detachment, high blood pressure, dural tap).
Fetal indications: fetal distress, failure to progress (malposition or malpresentation).
Lower-segment Caesarean section
Maternal indications: underlying maternal disease or pregnancy-related condition (e.g. placenta praevia, severe pre-eclampsia).
Fetal indications: fetal distress, failure to progress, malpresentation.
Congenital abnormality, severely compromised fetus (e.g. intrauterine growth restriction), risk of vertical transmission (HIV, primary genital herpes).

2   What are the conditions for attempting instrumental vaginal delivery?
Full dilatation, empty bladder, no head palpable per abdomen (maximum 1/5), position and station of the fetal head clearly identifiable, and adequate analgesia.

3   Compare and contrast Ventouse and forceps delivery.

Ventouse: less perineal trauma; less traction/detachment; increased failure rate and scalp trauma (cephalhaematoma).

Forceps: large diameter – hence more perineal trauma; need to define the exact position of the fetal head, especially if rotational forceps are used; facial nerve palsy; fracture of the skull; intracranial trauma possible; better success rate (better traction at delivery, and less maternal effort needed).

4   What are the maternal and fetal risks of operative delivery?

Maternal risks: bleeding; internal trauma; uterine rupture, especially with rotation; pain; long-term problems (e.g. incontinence, prolapse, dyspareunia).

Fetal risks: scalp lacerations; cephalhaematoma; sub-retinal haemorrhages; fracture of the skull; intracranial trauma (supratentorial tears, bleeding); facial nerve palsy.

5   What is a third-degree tear?

A perineal tear involving vaginal skin and perineal muscles and skin, including the anal sphincter, but intact rectal mucosa.

CORE PROBLEM 6: MINOR GYNAECOLOGICAL PROBLEMS

A 60-year-old woman has noticed 'dampness down below', together with some pruritus and dysuria.

Key topics

- Vulval tumours
- Urinary tract infection
- Urinary incontinence
- Prolapse

Vulval tumours

1   What are the cardinal features of vulval pruritus?

Itching and soreness of the vulva, especially at night. There may be associated redness, leukoplakia, excoriations, fissures and ulcerations.

2   How is vulval pruritus treated?

It depends on the cause: dermatosis (eczema, urticaria, contact allergies, psoriasis); infection (folliculitis, viral condylomata, *Candida*, *Trichomonas*, crab lice, scabies, pinworm); vulval dystrophies (lichen sclerosus); vulval intra-epithelial neoplasia, vulval carcinoma, poor hygiene, general medical conditions (diabetes, liver and renal impairment); psychogenic.

Treatment: remove the cause if possible. Adopt hygiene measures, avoid excessive heat, moisture, washing, use aqueous barrier creams, steroid cream, oestrogen cream, local anaesthetic cream and psychological support.

3   How is vulval cancer treated?
By radical vulvectomy and radiotherapy.

Urinary tract infection

1   What are the common symptoms and causative organisms?
Symptoms: dysuria, frequency, nocturia, incontinence, smelly urine, abdominal and loin pain, nausea, vomiting, haematuria, urinary retention.
Organisms: *E.coli*, *Pseudomonas*, *Klebsiella*, *Proteus*, *Streptococcus epiderdimidis*.

2   What are the predisposing factors for urinary tract infections?
Urinary stasis (renal stones, pregnancy, renal abnormalities, incomplete emptying), menopause, frequent sexual activity, catheterization (iatrogenic) and systemic disease (diabetes, neuropathic bladder).

Urinary incontinence

1   What are the different symptoms associated with incontinence?
Frequency, urgency, incontinence, stress incontinence, nocturia, incomplete emptying, double micturition and dysuria.

2   Differentiate between genuine stress incontinence (GSI) and detrusor instability (DI).
Stress and urge incontinence are symptoms, *NOT diagnoses*. These symptoms overlap. Genuine stress incontinence is incontinence with increased intra-abdominal pressure in the absence of detrusor contraction. Detrusor instability is incontinence due to involuntary detrusor contraction.

3   Why is urodynamics needed for diagnosis?
To distinguish between GSI and DI, as the treatment for these conditions is different. If urodynamics does not show any detrusor contractions, this can only be GSI. If detrusor contractions are present, this could be either DI or mixed DI and GSI .

4   What is the management of detrusor instability?
Bladder retraining drill and medical therapy (with anticholinergics and calcium antagonists).

5   What is the management of GSI?
Conservative: weight loss, pelvic floor exercises, vaginal cones, oestrogens.
Surgery: colposuspension (Burch, Marshall–Marchetti Kranz, Stamey, transvaginal tape, laparoscopic).

Prolapse

1   What are the risk factors for prolapse?
Age, parity, difficult childbirth (long second stage, big baby, instrumental delivery), increased intra-abdominal pressure (obesity, chronic cough, lifting) and menopause.

2   How is prolapse assessed clinically?
Pelvic examination in the supine, left lateral position with a Simm's speculum. Classified as anterior/mid/posterior compartment vs. first/second/third degree.

3   How can prolapse be treated?
Conservatively: weight loss, pelvic floor exercises, ring pessaries.
Surgery: anterior/posterior repair, vaginal hysterectomy, sacro-spinous fixation, abdominal sacro-colpopexy.

CORE PROBLEM 7: THE PROBLEM 14-YEAR-OLD

A father brings his 14-year-old daughter to the clinic. She is missing school because of regular 'tummy pains'.

Key topics

● Puberty
● Premenstrual syndrome
● Contraception
● Pelvic infection

Puberty

1   Describe how the hypothalamus controls ovulation.
GnRH-releasing factors from the hypothalamus enter the anterior pituitary via the hypophyseal portal system and stimulate secretion of FSH and LH (gonadotrophins). FSH and LH affect the ovarian cycle (follicular development and ovulation) and thus the secretion of ovarian hormones (oestrogen and progesterone). There is biofeedback of sex hormones on the pituitary and hypothalamus.

2   How do the normal secondary sex characteristics develop?
XX chromosomes are needed for normal ovarian development: 9–13 years, breast development; 9–14 years, pubic hair; 10–14 years, growth spurt; 11–15 years, menarche; 13–16 years, LH peak appears (ovulation and menses).

3   What are the proliferative and secretory menstrual phases?
They reflect changes in the endometrium during the menstrual cycle.
    The proliferative phase involves proliferation of endometrium from the basal layer under the influence of oestrogen.
    The secretory phase involves an increase in endometrial gland secretion and convolution under the influence of progesterone in preparation for implantation of a fertilized ovum.

4   What are the follicular and luteal ovarian phases?
They reflect changes in the ovary/follicle during the menstrual cycle.
    The follicular phase involves oocyte and follicular maturation. Oestradiol is produced with effects on the endometrium (proliferative phase).
    The luteal phase involves LH acting on granulosa cells to secrete progesterone. It corresponds to the secretory phase of the endometrium.

5   What anatomical abnormalities may this girl have?
Imperforate hymen, haematocolpos, haematometra, haematosalpinx.

Premenstrual syndrome

1   What are the common symptoms of premenstrual syndrome (PMS)?
Physical symptoms: fatigue, headaches, abdominal bloating, breast tenderness, swelling, acne, constipation.
Emotional symptoms: anxiety, hostility, anger, depression, tearfulness, irritability, over-sensitivity, panic attacks, loss of libido, inability to concentrate.
Behavioural symptoms: suicidal attempts, violence, disturbed interpersonal relationships, poor work performance.

2   Discuss the treatment options for PMS.
Hormonal: cyclical progesterones, combined oral contraceptive pill, GnRH, danazol, oestradiol.
Others: diuretics, vitamin B_6, evening primrose oil, antidepressants, psychotherapy, support; in extreme cases, hysterectomy and bilateral salpingo-oophorectomy (BSO).

Contraception

1   What is the Pearl index for various contraceptives?
The Pearl index is the number of unwanted pregnancies per 100 woman years.

Sterilization	0–1	IUCD	0.3–4
Mirena IUCD	0–1	Barrier	2–15
Combined oral contraceptive pill	0.1–1	Coitus interruptus	8–17
Progestogen-only pill	0.3–5	Rhythm method/ spermicidal agents	4–25

2   Compare hormonal with non-hormonal contraceptives.
Hormonal: anovulation, thickened cervical mucus, thin endometrium.
IUCD: prevents implantation, copper ions are toxic to sperm and zygote.
Barrier: reduce the risk of sexually transmitted diseases; some contain spermicidal agents.

3   What is emergency contraception?
Contraception after intercourse. It requires follow-up in case of failure.
Hormonal: prevention of ovulation and implantation. PC4 up to 72 hours after unprotected intercourse.
IUCD: prevents implantation, up to 7 days after ovulation.

4   What are the contraindications to the combined oral contraceptive pill?
Absolute: thrombophilia; history of deep-vein thrombosis/pulmonary embolus, previous cardiovascular accident; migraines; severe hypertension; oestrogen-dependent tumours; chronic liver disease; recent trophoblastic disease.
Relative: smoking; age; diabetes; sickle-cell disease.

Pelvic infection

1   What are the symptoms and signs of pelvic inflammatory disease (PID)?
Symptoms: pelvic pain, offensive discharge, abnormal vaginal bleeding, fever, dyspareunia, urological symptoms, nausea, vomiting.
Signs: pyrexia, abdominal tenderness, discharge, cervical excitation.

2   What are the common causes of PID and how are they treated?
Gonococcus (penicillins), *Chlamydia* (tetracyclines, erythromycin), bacterial vaginosis (metronidazole, clindamycin).

3   What is contact tracing?
Identification of any sexual contact, screening them for PID/sexually transmitted disease and treating them.

4   What is the differential diagnosis of PID?
Ectopic pregnancy, appendicitis, pyelonephritis, adnexal torsion, renal/biliary colic, endometriosis.

5   What are the short- and long-term complications of PID?

Short-term complications: tubo-ovarian abscess, sepsis, septic shock, disseminated intravascular coagulation.

Long-term complications: chronic PID, tubal damage/infertility, chronic pelvic pain, Fitz–Hugh–Curtis syndrome.

CORE PROBLEM 8: THE INFERTILE COUPLE

A couple have been 'trying for a baby' for 4 years. The woman is overweight and has painful, irregular periods.

Key topics

- Infertility
- Endometriosis
- Amenorrhoea
- Hirsutism

Infertility

1   What is the difference between primary and secondary infertility?

Infertility is failure to conceive after 12 months of trying for pregnancy.
   Primary: never pregnant before. Secondary: has had a previous pregnancy.

2   How is anovulation diagnosed and treated?

Irregular cycles suggest anovulation. It is investigated with day 21 progesterone, USS follicular tracking and LH surge detection in urine.

Ovulation induction drugs: clomiphene, human menopausal gonadotrophin, tamoxifen (risks include multiple pregnancy/ovarian hyper-stimulation syndrome) or surgery (ovarian drilling).

3   Discuss the risk factors for tubal occlusion, and the role of tubal surgery.

Risk factors include PID, previous surgery, endometriosis, bowel disease and appendicitis. Tubal surgery may have a role in some women, provided that the tubes are not damaged too much, but IVF is now a better and more successful option.

4   What do GIFT, ZIFT, IVF and ICSI stand for?

GIFT = gamete intra-Fallopian transfer. ZIFT = zygote intra-Fallopian transfer. IVF = *in vitro* fertilization. ICSI = intracytoplasmic sperm injection.

5   How is male factor infertility treated?

Obstructive azoospermia is treated by surgical reconstruction and sperm aspiration.

Testicular failure is treated by artificial donor insemination.
Oligospermia is treated by IVF with ICSI.
Erectile problems are treated by Viagra.

Endometriosis

1   What is the aetiology of endometriosis?
Retrograde menstruation, implantation, vascular/lymphatic embolism, transformation of peritoneal epithelium, immunological/genetic susceptibility.

2   List the common symptoms of endometriosis and the role of diagnostic
    laparoscopy.
Dysmenorrhoea, dyspareunia, cyclical pelvic pain, lower back pain, menstrual irregularity, infertility, chocolate cysts, cyclical rectal bleeding and haematuria. Diagnosis is made by laparoscopy.

3   Discuss the medical vs. surgical treatment of endometriosis.
Medical treatment: simulates pregnancy or menopause – oral contraceptive
    pill, continuous progestagens, danazol, GnRH analogues, Gestrinone.
Surgical treatment: laser, diathermy, excision (laparoscopic vs. open) and
    total abdominal hysterectomy with or without bilateral salpingo-
    oophorectomy.

4   What are chocolate cysts?
Endometriomas (endometriosis involving the ovaries).

Amenorrhoea

1   What is the definition of primary and secondary amenorrhoea?
Primary amenorrhoea is the non-appearance of menarche by the age of 16 years.
    Secondary amenorrhoea is the cessation of periods for more than 6 months.

2   What investigations would you perform for amenorrhoea?
Pregnancy test, FSH/LH, prolactin, thyroid function tests, androgen screen, chromosomes.
    Pelvic USS and possibly laparoscopy, bone age X-ray, MRI head.

3   Discuss the symptoms, investigations and treatment of polycystic ovary
    syndrome.
Symptoms: amenorrhoea, oligomenorrhoea, obesity, hirsutism, acne,
    infertility.
Investigations: LH/FSH on days 5–8 of cycle, androgen screen, prolactin.
    USS pelvis, enlarged smooth ovaries, 'pearl necklace'. Laparoscopy.

Treatment: weight loss, oral contraceptive pill to regulate cycle, treat hirsutism. Ovulation induction drugs (clomiphene, GnRH) or ovarian drilling.

4   Why should a pituitary tumour cause amenorrhoea?
Pituitary micro/macroadenomas secrete high levels of prolactin, which causes amenorrhoea.

Hirsutism

1   How would you investigate hirsutism?
History: familial or racial tendency.
Examination: hair body distribution, acne, weight, ovarian masses.
Investigations: androgens, FSH/ LH, prolactin, pelvic scan to exclude polycystic ovary syndrome, testosterone-secreting ovarian tumours.

2   What are the cosmetic and medical treatments for hirsutism?
Cosmetic: shaving, bleaching, waxing, electrolysis.
Medical: treat the cause (e.g. polycystic ovary syndrome, remove tumours), oral contraceptive pill (Dianette), cyproterone acetate.

CORE PROBLEM 9: THE MENOPAUSE

A 50-year-old woman has had increasingly heavy periods for 2 years.

Key topics

- Menorrhagia
- Menopause
- Gynaecological operations

Menorrhagia

1   What is dysfunctional uterine bleeding?
It is abnormal uterine bleeding in the absence of underlying organic pathology.
Menorrhagia is excess menstruation (> 80 mL).

2   What blood tests would you perform?
Full blood count, thyroid function tests, clotting.

3   Discuss the role of ultrasound and endometrial biopsy.
USS: endometrial thickness, ovarian morphology, contour of uterus.
Hysteroscopy: inspects endometrial cavity, with the option of direct sampling of endometrium.

4   Does every patient require an urgent hysteroscopy and D & C?
No, only women over 40 years of age require it to exclude intrauterine pathology.

5   What are the medical treatments for menorrhagia?
Hormonal treatments: oral contraceptive pill, danazol, GnRH, progestagens, Mirena IUCD.
Non-hormonal treatments: antifibrinolytics (tranexamic acid), non-steroidal anti-inflammatory drugs (mefenamic acid).

Menopause

1   What are the local/genital effects of the menopause?
Atrophy of the genital tract – atrophic vaginitis, postmenopausal bleeding, dyspareunia, vaginal dryness, urinary frequency, incontinence.

2   What are the distant/non-genital effects of the menopause?
Psychogenic – hot flushes, night sweats, mood swings, sleeplessness, lack of concentration, short-term memory loss, lack of libido.
Osteoporotic – hip fracture, vertebral fracture, Colles fracture.
Cardiovascular – ischaemic heart disease, cerebrovascular accident.

3   What routes of administration are available for HRT?
Oral, transdermal (patches, gel, creams, pessaries and implants).

4   What are the risks and benefits of HRT?
Benefits: relief of symptoms, reduction of risk of osteoporosis, ischaemic heart disease and cerebrovascular accident.
Risks: breast and endometrial cancer if unopposed E2 is used, thrombo-embolism.

Gynaecological operations

1   What are the various routes and types of hysterectomy?
Routes: vaginal, abdominal, laparoscopic.
Types: total and subtotal (cervix salvaged).

2   Compare abdominal with vaginal hysterectomy.
Abdominal: incision on the abdomen, easily accessible ovaries and other intra-abdominal organs.
Vaginal: no abdominal incision, less soreness, quicker recovery, often no access to ovaries, less easy to control bleeding.

3   What are the postoperative complications of hysterectomy?
Short-term complications: haemorrhage, infection (wound, pelvic, urinary tract infection, chest, phlebitis), thromboembolism.

Long-term complications: adhesions, ovarian failure, vault prolapse, psychological effects.

4   Does myomectomy have a role in the treatment of menorrhagia?
Yes, in women with fibroids who wish to retain their reproductive capability.

5   What are the advantages/disadvantages of endometrial ablation?
Advantages: day case, quick recovery, transcervical.
Disadvantages: only a 75% success rate at 5 years, small risk of hysterectomy.

CORE PROBLEM 10: HAVE I GOT CANCER?

A 65-year-old woman has had irregular vaginal bleeding for several weeks.

Key topics

- Cervical cancer
- Endometrial cancer
- Ovarian cancer
- Gynaecological operations

Cervical cancer

1   What are the major risk factors for cervical cancer?
Age, smoking, early age of sexual intercourse, multiple partners, human papilloma virus, cervical intra-epithelial neoplasia.

2   What is the difference between dyskaryosis and dysplasia?
Dyskaryosis is a cytological abnormality of the 'cell' (from a smear).
Dyplasia is a histological abnormality of a tissue (from a colposcopy/biopsy).

3   What colour are abnormal cells on colposcopy and why?
They are white. Acetic acid stains the abnormal cells which have a high protein content white. Iodine stains the normal cells which have a high glucose content brown.

4   How do we stage cervical cancer?
By clinical examination (vaginal examination) plus cystocopy and sigmoidoscopy. Stage 1 is confined to the cervix, stage 2 extends to the parametria and vaginal wall, stage 3 extends to the bladder/rectum and stage 4 has distant metastases.

Endometrial cancer

1   What are the risk factors for endometrial cancer?
Age, unopposed oestrogens, obesity, anovulatory cycles, polycystic ovary syndrome.

2   How is endometrial cancer staged?
Intra-operative and histological staging is used. Stage 1 is confined to the uterus, stage 2 extends to the ovaries/tubes/cervix, stage 3 extends to the bladder/rectum and stage 4 has distant metastases.

3   How is endometrial cancer treated?
Total abdominal hysterectomy/bilateral salpingo-oophorectomy, radiotherapy, hormonal treatment (Provera).

Ovarian cancer

1   Is screening for ovarian cancer routine?
No.

2   Why is the prognosis for ovarian cancer relatively poor?
Because it is often diagnosed at an advanced stage.

3   How is ovarian cancer staged?
By staging laparotomy. Stage 1 is confined to the ovaries, stage 2 is disease limited to the pelvis, stage 3 extends to the abdominal cavity/omentum and stage 4 has distant metastases.

4   What is the differential diagnosis of ovarian cysts in postmenopausal women?
Other tumours – fibroid, large bowel, endometrial or ovarian secondaries.

Gynaecological operations

1   Discuss the indications and complications of Wertheim's hysterectomy.
Indication: stage 1 and 2 carcinoma of the cervix.
Complications: bleeding, ureteric/vessel perioperative damage, infection, deep-vein thrombosis, lymphoedema, tumour recurrence or residual tumour left.

2   Would surgery be indicated even in advanced ovarian cancer?
Yes. Surgery is part of the staging process and it is important to get a tissue diagnosis. The primary surgical approach is debulking.

Index